MALE SEXUAL AWARENESS

MALE SEXUAL AWARENESS

Increasing Sexual Satisfaction

REVISED EDITION

BARRY & EMILY MCCARTHY

CARROLL & GRAF PUBLISHERS, INC.
NEW YORK

First Carroll & Graf edition 1988
Second edition 1998

Carroll & Graf Publishers, Inc.
19 W. 21st Street
New York, NY 10010

Library of Congress Cataloging-in-Publication Data

McCarthy, Barry W., 1943–
  Male sexual awareness / Barry & Emily McCarthy. — Rev. ed.
    p. cm.
  ISBN 0-7867-0473-X (alk. paper)
    1. Men—Sexual behavior.   2. Sex.   I. McCarthy, Emily J.
II. Title.
HQ28.M29   1998
306.7'081—dc21   97-45907
                                                               CIP

Manufactured in the United States of America

Contents

This book is dedicated to our grandson,
Torren Michael McCarthy,
with the hope that he and his generation
will enjoy an aware, responsible,
equitable, and pleasure-oriented approach
to sexuality.

MALE SEXUAL AWARENESS

1
MALE SEXUALITY—PERFORMANCE MACHINE
OR BEING A SEXUAL PERSON

Traditionally, men don't enroll in human sexuality courses, buy sexuality books, or ask sexual questions. If you are in a bookstore or find this book on a friend's coffee table, chances are you are feeling self-conscious. After all, men aren't supposed to read about sexuality, they're expected to know it all. Acknowledging there is something to learn is a sign of weakness, an admission you are not the super-confident, all-knowing, all-powerful man you are supposed to be.

It is a pity so many men feel this way because the present era is unparalleled in the amount of information that has been discovered about human sexuality. Surveys and laboratory studies have provided definitive answers to questions about sexual response and behavior that for years were matters of confusion and conflict. The investigations of Dr. Alfred Kinsey[1,2] (Source Notes in Appendix III) demonstrated the sexual activity of most of us was neither excessive nor unusual, but fit into a wide spectrum of normality. After Kinsey, it became clear everyone had a sex life, a fact that had been cast in doubt during the long sexual cover-up of the Victorian age. Another milestone came with the publications of Masters and Johnson[3,4]. Using an array of medical testing instruments as well as video recordings in a laboratory setting, these pioneering sex researchers studied the physiological responses of volunteers engaging in sexual intercourse and a variety of other sexual interactions. From this innovative investigation came a wealth of data on the ways in which people respond to sexual stimulation. With the birth of the sex therapy field in the 1970s, we've gained an understand-

1

ing of how to deal with sexual dysfunction and promote healthy functioning. In the 1980s and 1990s there has been a plethora of professional and public books on a variety of sexuality topics. The 1994 study, *Sex In America*[5], provided us with the clearest picture yet of attitudes, behavior, values, and feelings of a representative sample of American adults.

Courses on human sexuality from elementary school to high school from college to adult education have multiplied. Unfortunately, consumers of these books and courses have been women, not men. In Barry's college course "Human Sexual Behavior" there are 5 times more women enrolled. Male sexuality books are bought by women, not men. Women are more likely to seek therapy for a variety of individual, relationship, and family problems—the major exception is males are willing to seek therapy when there is a female sexual dysfunction (although resistant and avoidant if he has a sexual dysfunction, especially inhibited sexual desire). Males resist being seen as sexually unsure or vulnerable.

"But what does that have to do with me?" you ask. The answer is knowledge about human sexuality, especially male sexuality, is important to all of us. Although sexuality is a natural physiological function, sexual attitudes, behaviors, and emotional reactions are a result of complex learning and socialization. Our sexuality can be a source of great pleasure, a means of intimate communication, an expression of joy—or it can cause confusion, pain and unhappiness. Whether sex has a positive or negative effect depends at least in part on whether our sexual attitudes are based on ignorance and misinformation or on facts. Obtaining accurate information is the first step. Knowledge is power.

HOW MUCH DO YOU REALLY KNOW ABOUT MALE SEXUALITY?

Despite the advances in human sexuality, few of us are well informed about sex. Only one of six American men has received an adequate sex education. Despite the fact that the subject of sex permeates our society, sexual myths and misconceptions continue to dominate. Well informed, educated men accept beliefs about sexuality that are, in fact, untrue. If you wonder about your sexual knowledge, you might find it instructive to take the following test. Read each statement and indicate whether it is true or false. Don't worry about performance anxiety—it won't be graded.

1. The size of a man's penis is an indication of the strength of his sex drive.
2. The larger the penis, the greater the stimulation for the woman during intercourse.
3. A man's sexuality peaks during adolescence. After age twenty, sexual ability, interest, and enjoyment decline.
4. Men are interested in intercourse and orgasm. Affection and pleasuring appeal mostly to women.
5. The ability to ejaculate rapidly is a sign of masculinity.
6. If you fail to maintain an erection once, it is likely you will develop impotence.
7. Success in first intercourse is an indication of how successful he will be throughout his sexual life.
8. Black men have larger penises than white men and a stronger sex drive.
9. Masturbation is detrimental to a man's sexual ability.
10. Enjoying giving oral-genital sex is a sign of immaturity and insecurity.
11. Male and female sexual interests and responses are essentially different.
12. Having fantasies or feelings of attraction for men is a sign of homosexuality.
13. Homosexuality is a form of mental illness.
14. The most natural position for sexual intercourse is male on top.
15. A healthy, well-adjusted man should have no trouble performing sexually in any situation.
16. Since conception takes place in the woman's body, it is her responsibility to prevent an unwanted pregnancy.
17. Erection is always a sign of sexual excitement and a need for intercourse.
18. A good lover is able to give his partner an orgasm each time they have intercourse.
19. Some men are naturally better lovers. While you may be able to learn certain sexual skills, you will never match the performance of someone who has more innate ability.

20. Simultaneous orgasm is the most fulfilling sexual goal for a couple.
21. The normal frequency of intercourse for a couple in their twenties or early thirties is four times a week. Having intercourse less often indicates a low sex drive.
22. Sexual intercourse should be avoided during menstruation and pregnancy.
23. Men who have suffered a heart attack or stroke should avoid intercourse.
24. Women transmit the HIV virus to men twice as much as men transmit HIV to women.
25. When a man reaches adulthood, he loses interest in fantasy and masturbation.

If you answered true for any of these statements, there are things you can learn about sexuality, because every one is false. These are common sex myths, many of which are widely accepted despite overwhelming scientific evidence to the contrary. They have led to incalculable dissatisfaction, frustration, insecurity, and misunderstanding for both men and women.

MALE RESISTANCE TO SEXUAL KNOWLEDGE

Inaccurate sexual information is detrimental to both men and women. Yet it is men who perpetuate and cling to the old sex myths. Because men are expected to be sexual experts, it is difficult to suggest they might be wrong or misinformed. Because they cannot admit ignorance, they will not ask questions or be receptive to new sexual understandings. The old and damaging sex myths are perpetuated *ad infinitum*, as well as new myths being generated.

One paradox about sexuality in this generation is the people wisest about sex aren't men but women. Women are far more open to sexual information and advice. They are willing to admit lack of knowledge and expertise, while men are convinced what we don't know isn't worth learning. Women are aware there is room for change, growth, and increased satisfaction.

Walk into any bookstore or library and look at the books on sexuality. You will see many volumes for, by, and about women, but few devoted to male sexuality. The receptivity of women to self-help advice is well known. Publishers assume (and not without reason) that men will turn away from such books with a shrug of "Who needs it? I know more than these people." The majority of books on male sexuality are bought and read by women.

It is not only in bookstores that one sees evidence of the male know-it-all attitude toward sex. Barry has encountered it many times in his work as a psychology professor. For twenty-seven years he's taught a course in human sexual behavior at a large metropolitan university. Not only do five times as many female students enroll in the course, but males ask fewer questions and rarely take part in class discussions. Female students are no more embarrassed to reveal their incomplete knowledge of human sexuality than they would be to confess ignorance of organic chemistry or English literature. As a result, they derive far greater benefit.

RELUCTANCE TO DISCUSS SEXUALITY

This reluctance to learn about sex from books or in classroom situations extends to exchanging sexual information or discussing sexual feelings on a personal basis. Few fathers are able to communicate freely with their sons (or daughters) about sexuality. Far too often, sex is a taboo subject in the home until the father finally decides it is time to inform his son about the "facts of life" or give him a package of condoms and tell him to stay out of trouble. This father-son confrontation takes the form of a brief, awkward lecture that answers only such basic questions as who puts what where, if even that. Since the father himself harbors many misconceptions, he is likely to pass sex misinformation and harmful attitudes on to his son. Moreover, since the son has been discouraged from thinking of his parents as sexual people, and he senses his father's discomfort, he is unwilling to ask questions or ask advice. He, like his father, pretends to be knowledgeable and experienced.

The reluctance to discuss sex frankly and openly affects other male relationships. It is rare to find young males who are truthful with each other about sexual experiences, especially first intercourse. The best available statistics indicate 25 percent of males are unsuccessful in their first intercourse because they ejaculate before the penis enters the vagina or are so anxious they don't get or can't keep an erection. One out of four is a substantial proportion, enough to make the experience very common. And yet, can you imagine the following dialogue?

"Hey, Jim, how'd it go with Stephanie last night?"

"Not good, Gordon. I came before I could get in."

"Well, don't worry, Jim. You'll improve with practice and gain confidence."

It is far more likely Jim would claim he had performed like a prize bull, even if it had been the fiasco of his young life. He would claim Stephanie was so impressed she'd pay him to have sex with her. Or, if Jim were so foolish as to admit he had an erection or early ejaculation problem, Gordon would never let him hear the end of it. We are not kind to each other where sex is concerned. People who harbor anxieties and insecurities rarely are.

LIVING UP TO MALE PERFORMANCE DEMANDS

Men cheat themselves out of sexual pleasure. Not only are we expected to be sexually knowledgeable without having received adequate instruction, but are expected to perform flawlessly at every opportunity. Trying to live up to these impossible demands causes anxiety and insecurity. For men, sex is a bluff, a desperate struggle to maintain the image of the infallible "male performance machine." When sex is so competitive, so performance oriented, there is little room for pleasure. Sex is what you do to a woman to prove something to her or yourself. Sex is not supposed to be comfortable, intimate, sharing or pleasurable.

The size of our equipment, the number of times we can come—these are the things that concern us, not how much pleasure we give and receive. Most destructive is the notion that we must never default, never fail to perform. According to the commonly accepted mythical standard, a "real man is willing and able to have sex anytime, anywhere, with any woman." It doesn't occur to us that the ability to meet such demands is simply not human. Absolute reliability is a standard that should be applied to machines, not people. And yet, this is precisely what we demand of ourselves sexually.

Women have begun sloughing off their rigid, inhibited, sexual socialization. Men can learn a great deal from their example. The goal of the feminist movement is not to put down men but to alter the confining and rigid roles that frustrate both men and women. Women have an awakened sense of themselves as autonomous beings, in control of and responsible for their wellbeing and sexuality. It is a shame when men feel threatened by women who insist on equity as people and sex partners. The most satisfying sexual experiences result when both the man and woman are aware of and express their sexual needs and preferences as well as respond to those of their partner. When each person is sexually aware and feels responsible for his/her sexuality, it facilitates being an intimate team and a mutually satisfying sexual relationship.

Our goal is not to transform the man into a super-lover whose performance will leave his partners panting for more. Understanding a woman's anatomy, her pattern of receptivity, and knowing the kinds of stimulation that are most effective in producing arousal and orgasm are necessary aspects of being a good lover, but not the most important. A sensitive lover is not a technician; he is someone who can enjoy and be involved in feelings of tenderness, intimacy, eroticism and emotional expression that occur during sex. In addition to knowing how to give pleasure, he is able to accept it as well. He feels deserving of pleasure. He understands lovemaking is not just a skill to be practiced within the confines of the bedroom, but is an expression of feelings of comfort, affection, pleasure, and eroticism. He realizes sexuality is more than his penis, intercourse, and orgasm—it is a positive integral part of being a man. He wants sexuality to enhance his life and intimate relationships, not cause anxiety, confusion, guilt, or trauma.

WHAT THIS BOOK IS ABOUT

The focus of this book is twofold. First, to present the most accurate, reliable information presently available on male sexuality and topics related to sexual functioning. Second, to help men integrate their sexuality with the rest of their lives in a way that enhances awareness and satisfaction. Sex *per se* is limited to genitals, intercourse, and orgasm while sexuality involves the whole range of attitudes, behaviors, and emotions concerning you, masculinity, intimacy, and sexual expression. This book is addressed to men, but women are encouraged to read it as well.

Indeed, since sexuality is the most intimate form of human communication, it can be extremely beneficial for a woman to gain insight into the needs and conflicts that affect her man.

This book is comprehensive in covering a wide variety of issues of interest and importance to men. You can read the chapters consecutively, as a survey of male sexuality, or use the book as a reference source to be consulted about specific issues and problems. The book is divided into three sections: (1) facts to increase your knowledge and help you own your sexuality; (2) ways to enhance your sexuality; and (3) dealing with problems and issues that interfere with sexual satisfaction. Where there is a question of sexual values, we advocate positions on the basis of Barry's expertise as a practicing psychologist, sex therapist, and professor of psychology as well as our personal and couple experiences. You need to take into account your background, experiences, and values in deciding how relevant our recommendations are to your life. The range of normal sexual behavior takes in any private activity between consenting adults that involves sharing and pleasure, is not coercive, does not involve children, and is not physically or psychologically destructive. The choice is yours, depending on what you and your partner find pleasurable and satisfying.

A PERSONAL NOTE

Writing and revising this book has been a challenging and rewarding experience. The first edition in 1988 was written solely by Barry. Since then we have coauthored five books, *Sexual Awareness, Female Sexual Awareness, Couple Sexual Awareness, Intimate Marriage,* and *Confronting the Victim Role.* Working together on this book has provided a balanced view of male sexuality. This will enhance its value for both male and female readers. Relationships based on respect, trust, intimacy, and equity, which is our value position, enhance emotional and sexual satisfaction.

Barry's preparation for writing about male sexuality has included not only formal training and study in the fields of psychology and human sexuality but many of the experiences, both negative and positive, that form the background of males in our society. Growing up in Chicago in the 1950s, he received no real sex education from family, church, or school. What knowledge he had came largely from peers, and if, as a young man, he had taken the sex-myth quiz presented earlier, he would have done poorly. Like most of his friends, he thought of sex in terms of conquest and performance. Although he managed to "score" with women, his achievements never seemed quite up to par, and he invariably exaggerated them. He took little responsibility in these early encounters, leaving contraception to the woman and sexually transmitted diseases to luck. Nor did it occur to him to care about or even notice the woman's responses. When he was twenty-one, he began an affair that lasted a year and a half. This was the first time he related to a sex partner on a person-to-person basis—an important learning experience.

At the age of twenty-two, he started graduate work in psychology at Southern Illinois University. It was there that Barry and Emily met, and were married a year later. Emily's experiences growing up in a small factory town outside Peoria were quite different than Barry's. Her sexual socialization focused on the traditional female fear of becoming pregnant and that derailing her life. Her mother and two older brothers were quite protective—Emily was the first of her family to go to college. Throughout high school and college she was very social, but sexually reserved. For Emily, sexuality was closely associated with a serious relationship. We were a good example of traditional double-standard sexual socialization.

Despite the closeness and affection we felt for each other, we carried into the marriage many erroneous and destructive assumptions about sex and sex roles. This caused problems and conflicts that had to be confronted if we were to achieve intimacy and sexual satisfaction. Although we did not have a sexual dysfunction, our sexual life was mediocre. Sex was high frequency, but low quality. It took well over a year before we were able to communicate, experiment, and develop a comfortable, functional, couple sexual style. Today, after thirty years of marriage and three children (two biological, one adopted), and one grandchild, sex continues to be a high-quality, integral part of our marital bond. We attribute this not only to the fact that we respect and care deeply about each other but also to the accurate sexual information and positive attitudes we've developed. We are committed to integrate sexual awareness into our lives and marriage.

Barry's decision to go into the field of sex therapy came about, as such decisions often do, quite accidentally. He chose a research project in sexual dysfunction, and found, to his surprise, that in 1969 there had been very little work done in that field. This aroused his interest and eventually led him to teaching courses in human sexuality and focusing his clinical work on sexual problems. Barry became a certified marital and sex therapist. Sexual problems are a result of poor learning experiences and a lack of respectful communication. Sexual functioning and satisfaction can be improved by gaining better understanding, developing an aware, positive attitude toward sexuality, and viewing sexual intimacy as a shared pleasure. Integral to this is treating the woman, whether a spouse or dating partner, in a respectful, cooperative, and equitable manner.

Being male is not something you should be ashamed of or apologetic about. We do not believe men, either individually or as a group, have to atone for the sins of male chauvinism. No amount of guilt, shame, or apologies will cause a relationship to become more satisfying. In fact, it's counterproductive for intimacy and sexuality. What is needed is not guilt, but understanding, sensitivity, and a commitment to change in the present and future. When these are achieved, there is no limit to the pleasure, satisfaction, and security that can be derived from an intimate sexual relationship.

In the following chapters we will be dealing with topics relating to the male sexual life cycle, methods of enhancing sexual self-esteem and functioning, choices and responsibilities that are a necessary part of your sexuality, and dealing with problems that inhibit the full expression of sexuality. Throughout, we draw on case studies of clients Barry has treated (their identities have been disguised), as well as our personal experiences, to provide relevant illustrations of the points discussed.

This is a book of ideas and information, not a do-it-yourself therapy book or a treatise on sexual techniques. If, by presenting an integrated and positive view of male sexuality, our book can help you reexamine your attitudes and gain the intimate satisfactions male performance myths have cheated you out of, we will be satisfied. We hope this book will be helpful to you and those you care about and who care about you.

2
A GUIDE TO YOUR BODY AND ITS
SEXUAL CAPACITY

From the moment we are born, we are fascinated by our bodies. Within the first year, we can produce pleasurable sensations by rubbing and stroking our genitals: sexual awareness is born. Awareness grows as we mature. Not only is it natural for young children to touch themselves, it is natural to be intensely curious about their sex organs—and those of others. Examining and comparing genitals, mutual genital touching, playing "house" or "doctor"—these activities are part of normal development. Looking, touching, and exploring are important in developing healthy attitudes toward your body and sexuality.

Unfortunately, as children, we received strong messages of disapproval that discouraged us from pursuing body exploration. We learned our bodies, especially our genitals, were something to be hidden, to be ashamed of. Some parents go so far as to teach children to avoid looking at their bodies. As a result of these messages, our natural curiosity is blunted. As adults, we tell ourselves the time for self-exploration is over, we have outgrown such childish pursuits, there is nothing left to learn. Actually, the average adult knows surprisingly little about his body in general and his genitals specifically. This stance of detached indifference detracts from your capacity to feel comfortable with your body and enjoy your sexuality.

GENITAL EXPLORATION AND AWARENESS
We encourage you to give way to long-suppressed curiosity and become acquainted with your body. Find a time when you

11

have at least thirty minutes of privacy—it could be the next time you take a bath or shower—and set it aside for sexual self-exploration. Take off your clothes and sit on the bed or the floor. A full-length mirror would be helpful because it gives you a more complete view. You may want to use a hand mirror to look at hard to see areas. Relax and put aside any thought that you are doing something unnatural or unhealthy. You are taking a good look at your body, and who has a better right to do that than you?

Start with the testicles (or balls, if you prefer—you can use proper or slang words). Hold them in your hand, using the hand mirror to examine them from all sides. Be aware of their weight and shape. You needn't be afraid of hurting them. We know how painful a low blow can be, but under normal circumstances, the testicles are surprisingly resilient. Our dependence on athletic supporters for protection during strenuous activities is a learned need. Male animals, whose testicles are no less vulnerable than ours, engage in physical activities that make human athletics seem tame, and yet suffer no ill effects. Among primitive peoples, males run, dance, and fight without wearing supporters, and seldom experience genital injury.

The testicles are the principal male sex glands. Inside the two egg-shaped bodies are the *seminiferous tubules*, glands within which sperm are manufactured. The testicles manufacture the sex hormone, testosterone, which is responsible for triggering the development of male physical characteristics. Testosterone is the hormone which most effects sexual desire. So efficient are the testicles in maintaining a satisfactory testosterone level that if one is removed, the remaining testicle is capable of carrying on by itself without any decrease in sexual or procreative functioning.

If you have medical questions about sexual functioning—hormonal, vascular or neurological—the physician of choice is a urologist or someone with a speciality in sexual medicine. The urologist is the closest thing to a gynecologist for men. Men are encouraged to do monthly testicle self-examination to ensure early detection of testicular cancer (this is similar to the female's self-examination for breast cancer). The male can examine his testicles after a hot bath or shower to determine whether there are small, hard lumps that could be tumors. If you detect something amiss, immediately consult your general physician or a urologist.

Sperm are created by the millions in the testicles. The sperm travel through the *epididymis* where they become mature. Sperm leave the testicles by way of the *vas deferens,* two soft, thin tubes which go into the body cavity. The vas leads into the seminal vesicles, storage chambers for the sperm, and then into the prostate. It is in the *prostate* that the sperm are mixed with seminal fluid, the whitish alkaline liquid that spurts from the penis during ejaculation. Sperm are extremely tiny, contributing only slightly to the total volume of the ejaculate, the major portion (97 percent) of which consists of seminal fluid (semen). Thus, when the vas deferens is severed in the vasectomy operation, only sperm are left out of the mix. A sterilized male continues to ejaculate semen as before, with no decrease in force, amount or enjoyment.

The testicles are housed in a bag of loose, wrinkled skin called the scrotum. One testicle usually hangs lower than the other. The scrotum can contract or relax, at times allowing the testicles to dangle freely against the thighs, at other times drawing them up into a neat, tight package. These changes correspond to a rise or fall in temperature. In order to manufacture sperm, the testicles must be a few degrees cooler than normal body temperature. The scrotum's ability to contract is a device for regulating internal temperature. When it is cold the muscles contract, warming the testicles by bringing them in close contact with the body. When the outside temperature rises, the opposite occurs, and the testicles are repositioned to cool them off.

The scrotal muscles come into play during sexual excitement. When aroused, a man's testicles rise in the scrotum and increase in size. If arousal does not culminate in ejaculation, the swelling remains, causing an uncomfortable condition popularly known as "blue balls," i.e., prolonged vasocongestion. This is temporary, however, and causes no damage.

Physiologically, there are three systems which must be in place to enable sexual functioning—hormonal, vascular and neurological. Popular culture emphasizes male sexual performance is strongest between 18 and 21 when the main hormones are activated and he is at the peak of his physical functioning. What a self-defeating message to give a man that sexually he's over the hill at 21. It is true there are fewer professional athletes after age 30, and almost none after age 40. That's because your hormonal, vascular, and neurological systems function less efficiently. However, sex is not an athletic performance—you are not competing for a gold medal for quickest erections and orgasms. At its base, sexuality is about giving and receiving pleasure. You become less of a sexual athlete with age, but can be a more sensitive lover. Sexuality is about sharing pleasure, not giving an "A" performance. You want to practice healthy eating, exercise, sleeping, not smoking, and moderate drinking since good health facilitates sexuality. Your hormonal, vascular, and neurological systems need to be functional, but you do not need to be a perfect, high performance machine.

EXPLORING YOUR PENIS

Emerging just above the scrotum is the base of the penis. There are very few men who have not handled and looked at their penis. It is the focus of intense emotions; few men regard their penis dispassionately. You may be proud of it, ashamed of it, anxious about it, afraid of it, or have mixed feelings about it, but it is unlikely you think of your penis with the same attitude you have, for example, toward your ear. Yet the penis is an organ like any other.

It is worthwhile to clear your mind of preconceived notions and look at your penis as if you have never seen it before. The penis is composed chiefly of spongy tissue! There are three distinct cylindrical bodies, two on top and one underneath, which are bound together by sheets of thin membrane. Erection occurs when blood enters the penis through arteries running through the erectile tissue. Simultaneously, muscles near the base of the penis contract, preventing blood from leaving the penis. Erection is triggered by nerve centers in the lower spinal column. The actual stimulus may come from the brain in the form of erotic thoughts or anticipation, or from direct tactile stimulation. The first kind of erection, called "spontaneous" or "automatic," is common in younger men. As men become older, they need more penile stroking and stimulation. This is not an indication they are developing a problem—it means the pattern of sexual response gradually changes with age. Erectile dysfunction is a different problem and is *not* a normal consequence of aging. Sex becomes more intimate and interactive. The more the man is aware and accepting of normal bodily changes, the better his sexual functioning.

Erection is a natural physiological response. A newborn male baby has his first erection within a few minutes of delivery. Every night while sleeping, whether sexually active or not, the male has an erection every ninety minutes, thus having three to five erections during the night. Laboratory studies have been done with ninety-year-old men in good health who have erections and function sexually. You are truly a sexual person from the day you're born to the day you die.

The head of the penis is called the glans. This is the most sensitive part of the penis, containing an extremely high concentration of nerve endings. The most sensitive area of the glans is the ridge at its base, called the corona. On the underside of the penis, where the corona divides into a sort of swallowtail shape, there is a small flange of skin joining the glans to the shaft, which is highly sensitive. The areas of greatest sensitivity vary according to the individual. Some men, for example, may find the shaft of their penis particularly responsive to stimulation. Some enjoy having their anal area stimulated, while others find this not at all pleasurable. In uncircumcised men, the foreskin, or prepuce, extends over the glans but retracts when the penis becomes erect. Jews, Muslims, and many other ethnic and religious groups remove the foreskin in an operation known as circumcision. Circumcision has become a common practice in many advanced nations, but for health reasons rather than religious or cultural ones. The oily substance emitted by the Tyson's glands, located just behind the corona, collects under the uncircumcised foreskin to form a smelly deposit called smegma. Smegma can be eliminated by regular cleaning, but when it is not, it may become a source of infection. Opponents of circumcision maintain removal of the foreskin renders a man less sensitive to sexual stimulation and reduces his enjoyment. But, it is in the glans and not the foreskin that the concentration of nerve endings is highest. Anyone who feels his capacity for arousal is not what it should be is wasting time if he tries to pin the blame on the physician who performed the circumcision.

THE MYTH OF PENIS SIZE

One reason to get our facts straight about male sexual anatomy and physiology is that this area has been obscured by superstition and misinformation. Men who readily accept scientific findings in other fields stubbornly perpetuate myths about the penis as though a loyalty to self-defeating sexual folklore is a prerequisite of being a "real man." The myth that continues to exert a powerful negative influence in the face of scientifically established fact concerns penis size. To eliminate the destructive effects of the penis size myth, let us discuss this in detail.

Penis size differences (or imagined differences) have been the basis for an enormous amount of male anxiety. Perhaps the sense of inadequacy has its roots in the childhood experience of a young boy comparing his father's penis with his own. To a child, an adult penis may seem so large and formidable that he cannot imagine ever growing to that size. Once a feeling of inadequacy takes root, it is easily reinforced. One way this occurs is making comparisons between your penis and those of other males, often in the world of the locker room. What male has not found himself glancing (surreptitiously, of course, so as not to be mistaken for having a homosexual interest) at the genitals of other men as they change into swimsuits or gym shorts and finding nearly all of them seem larger than his?

Such a comparison is misleading for two reasons. First, as the result of perspective, a penis looks larger when seen from a distance as part of someone else's body than seen from above as part of one's own. Second, it is misleading to judge the size of a penis when it is in the flaccid state. The larger a man's penis when limp, the less it will increase in size when erect. Penises which are smaller in the flaccid state have a greater erectile potential. Thus, there is an equalizing factor. Variations in size among erect penises are minimal.

There are individual variations in penis size, of course, just as there are variations in body size. However, penis length varies much less than body height (nor are height and penis size related). The average penis is from two and a half to four inches long in the flaccid state and from five and a half to six and a half inches long when erect, with a diameter of about one inch flaccid and about one and a half inches when erect. But these are only averages, and, like most averages, do not mean much, except perhaps that someone, somewhere, has been very busy with a measuring tape. It would be more meaningful to say a normal penis is of proper size to function in intercourse. This definition takes in just about all men. Interestingly, 2 of 3 men believe their penis is smaller than average. Other than being an obvious statistical anomaly, it demonstrates how the performance machine orientation to sex predisposes men to be anxious and insecure. Psychological well-being is promoted by adopting a positive body image, which includes acceptance of your penis and sexuality.

The myth that men with larger penises have a stronger sex drive and are capable of greater sexual performance is tenacious. The reasoning is that the larger a man's muscles, the stronger he is. However, as anyone who has taken a course in elementary logic knows, analogy can be a highly misleading form of reasoning. The speciousness of this idea becomes clear when we examine the results of controlled, scientific studies. Masters and Johnson observed the sexual functioning of hundreds of subjects under laboratory conditions. They found no relationship whatever between penis size and sexual desire or functioning.

The related idea that a large penis is capable of giving a woman more pleasure is based on the mistaken notion that it is the vagina which is the source of a woman's sexual response. Actually, a woman's most sensitive genital organ is the clitoris— a small, cylindrical organ located at the top of the vestibule at the joining of the labia minora. The clitoris has, in fact, fully as many nerve endings as the glans of the penis, concentrated into a much smaller area. It is the focal point of female sexual pleasure, just as the glans of the penis is the focal point for the male. During intercourse, the clitoris is stimulated by pulling and rubbing action caused by pelvic thrusting—stimulation that is independent of penis size. The vagina, which is in direct contact with the penis, has fewer nerve endings, most of which are in the outer third. Moreover, the vagina is an active rather than passive organ and can adjust to the penis whatever its size. Sexual incompatibility based on the size of a couple's genitals is, with extremely rare exceptions, a myth.

Because of the distendible nature of the vagina, virtually any man and woman are well suited, at least physically, to give each other pleasure during intercourse. Sexual attraction, desire, and functioning are based on much more than genitals. In fact, they are not based on genitals at all.

It is true some women may be attracted to men with large penises in much the same way some men are attracted to women with large breasts. Pornographic films, magazines, and books—with their emphasis on physical endowments—are at least partially to blame for encouraging an obsession (more for anxious men—women typically do not emphasize penis size) with men who are ''hung,'' just as they encourage a male obsession with women who are ''stacked.'' This reinforces feelings of inadequacy among men and women who think they are smaller than average. But, as we have seen, a woman who imagines that a large penis automatically makes a man an excellent lover is just as naive as a man who believes all large-breasted women are aroused through breast stimulation. A passion for size on the part of either a man or a woman is a bias, and, as such, is her personal concern. Why let someone else's misconceptions serve as a criterion for your sexual self-esteem?

LEARNING TO BE A SEXUAL LOVER

In the last analysis, whatever nature has given us is ours to make the most of. Nor do we have cause to accuse nature of favoring some men over others. With rare exceptions, we are equally suited physically to both give and receive sexual pleasure. Lovers are made, not born. Your ability to enjoy sex and to make sex enjoyable for your partner is dependent on your comfort, awareness, skill, sensitivity, imagination, and ability to communicate—all of which are a matter of learning and experience. Once a man becomes aware of his potential as a lover and learns how truly satisfying his sex life can be if he gives up performance-oriented sex for pleasure-oriented sex, the question of size can be forgotten.

3
CONTRACEPTION AND VASECTOMY: PLANNED, WANTED CHILDREN

Sex functions as a shared pleasure, a means to reinforce intimacy, and a tension reducer. Traditionalists object to our pleasure-oriented concept, emphasizing the biological purpose of sex for reproduction.

Historically, people believed reproduction was the sole purpose of sex. Sexual pleasure was the prize nature offered men for producing children. If this prize did not exist, if each couple had to reproduce in a rational, deliberate, and mechanical way, it is unlikely the human race would be facing its present crisis of overpopulation.

Sex has accomplished the task of preserving the human race much too well. In our advanced society, where widely available medical facilities ensure nearly all children will survive to reproductive age, the biological function of sex presents a serious problem. Couples who pursue sexual pleasure without thought for the consequences produce more offspring than they can afford to house, clothe, and feed. Society is then burdened with the care of these children, or they become victims of poverty and neglect.

The answer is family planning, specifically the use of contraceptives. Contraception disconnects sex from procreation, allowing them to be what they should be—separate activities for separate purposes. Contraception makes it possible to enjoy sexual pleasure without producing unplanned, unwanted children. Effective contraceptive devices are one of our greatest technological achievements, a significant victory in people's struggle to make rational, healthy decisions and control their lives.

ATTITUDES TOWARD CONTRACEPTION

The male attitude toward birth control is misguided and unfortunate. Many men, particularly those who are single, think of contraception as primarily, or solely, a female concern. The male attitude toward contraception is characterized by aversion. This is particularly evident when the birth control method is the one for which he is responsible. "Why wear a raincoat in the shower?" typifies a man's response to the suggestion he use a condom. The specious logic breaks down under rational analysis: wearing a raincoat would be a very sensible precaution if the consequences of showering in the nude were as negative as an unwanted pregnancy (or a sexually transmitted disease or contracting the HIV virus).

Why are so many of us reluctant or unwilling to assume responsibility for contraception? In part, the answer relates to exploitative masculine attitudes that form the basis of the double standard. If sex is something men get from women under false pretenses, then the male has no responsibility for the consequences of his actions. Sex is the man's domain, contraception is the woman's domain.

The "macho" ideal leaves no room for men to feel responsible for conception, contraception or children. Instead, we play the role of the uncommitted, sexually driven male with no thought for negative consequences. This creates a psychological bind. While normal human concern and simple common sense make us want to take precautions against an unwanted pregnancy, the masculine code counsels us to "take sexual risks, only wimps fear consequences." Asking the woman whether she was protected contraceptively is antithetical to the romantic, seductive scenario.

Distorted notions of reproduction are another factor in men's disregard of birth control. Because pregnancy occurs within the woman's body, the responsibility for preventing conception is construed as lying entirely with her. Pregnancy is an inherent weakness of female biology. Pregnancy is a feminine worry, especially in premarital sex. The logical flaw here is that while pregnancy may indeed be a condition exclusive to women, conception is not. Intercourse occurs, or should occur, by mutual consent. Conception occurs when a male sperm and a female egg, each containing half the number of chromosomes needed to create a human life, merge and grow into a fetus. Wherever the embryo may actually grow, the responsibility for triggering its development lies equally with the man and woman—as does the responsibility for preventing conception.

Even if the woman tells you it is all right to have intercourse without using anything, you are not absolved of responsibility. There is a great deal of ignorance about fertility among women. The majority of women do not ovulate on a regular twenty-eight-day cycle, so the most likely outcome of relying on the rhythm method, i.e., trying to time intercourse for when she is not about to ovulate, is an unwanted pregnancy. At any given intercourse, the probability of conception is less than five percent. However, a couple who are regularly having intercourse without contraception run a 75 percent probability of becoming pregnant within 6 months.

Another reason for the prevailing male attitude stems from the erroneous connection between masculinity and the ability to sire children. If a man believes impregnating a woman is a way of demonstrating his virility, he may secretly welcome a pregnancy. Actually, there is no correspondence between sexual ability and capacity to procreate. Conception depends on his sperm count and motility, which has no effect on either sex drive or sexual skill. A man may be a great lover and be sterile, or he can be quite fertile yet sexually dysfunctional. By the way, many males prefer having a male child and blame the woman if they continue to have daughters. In truth, it is the male sperm that determines whether the baby will be male or female.

THE MYTH OF SPONTANEOUS, ROMANTIC SEX

Some men avoid taking responsibility for contraception because they feel that to introduce this subject will destroy the romantic mood they are counting on to sweep away the partner's hesitancies about intercourse. The woman is often guilty of complicity, for she too wishes to preserve the fiction they are so carried away by sexual excitement they are unable to stop for something so mundane as a contraceptive device. Such self-deception is especially common in first intercourse situations, where excitement and anxiety are pronounced. Less than one-third of couples engaging in intercourse for the first time use effective contraception. A helpful guideline is if the couple are not ready to talk about having sex and using contraception, they have no business having intercourse.

The couple do not perceive their lack of common-sense precaution as a result of guilt and confusion about sexuality. They act according to the romantic myth that sex is best when spontaneous. Certainly romanticism and spontaneity add to the enjoyment of sex. But spontaneity and planning are not mutually exclusive. An unwanted pregnancy is far too high a price to pay for the preservation of romantic illusions, but many pay this price. One of three women has an unplanned premarital pregnancy. One in four women is pregnant at time of marriage or have a child (for teenage marriages it is more than three of four). The United States has one of the highest rates of unplanned pregnancies among developed countries. If a couple is not able to make a decision to use effective contraception, they are not ready to engage in intercourse.

ACTING RESPONSIBLY

Once you've become convinced to assume your share of the responsibility for contraception, how do you go about putting that conviction into practice? It may not be easy, particularly for a single man. A couple's decision to have sex is most often expressed not in verbal terms but in a language of glances, signs, and body language. "One thing led to another, and we found ourselves in bed," expresses the experience of many couples. This is especially true when alcohol or drugs are involved. The problem is how to interrupt that nonverbal and highly enjoyable sequence by discussing birth control, without destroying the sexual mood.

A common fear is your partner will think less of you for bringing up a prosaic subject such as contraception while in the heat of passion, she'll see you as overcautious and unromantic. It is unlikely she'll react that way. After all, it is she who is in danger of becoming pregnant, so precautions taken to prevent pregnancy are in her interest. She will take your concern as a sign you are interested in her welfare. Rather than eliciting scorn, discussing contraception will cause her to see you as a responsible and caring lover.

It is true, though, that bringing up the subject of contraception can break the romantic mood. The more frankly the subject is introduced, the less of an intrusion it will be. Ask straightforwardly whether she is protected by the pill, Depo-Provera injections, Norplant, an IUD, or a diaphragm. Assuming both partners are aware of what they are doing, a note of realism, introduced in good faith, should not present an obstacle for either the man or the woman.

MALE CONTRACEPTIVES

Another solution is for the man to provide contraception himself. Of the contraceptive methods available, only two are male-oriented—the condom and vasectomy. The preponderance of female-centered contraceptive methods reflects the attitude of our society that contraception is the female's responsibility. Contraceptive research focuses on devices involving the female, and this is unlikely to change in the near future. There has been research on a birth control pill for men and an injection which would cause sterility for a period of months. Urologists had talked of a reversible vasectomy in which a valve is installed in the vas deferens to turn the flow of sperm on and off. However, there are technical problems with these devices as well as concerns over physical and sexual side effects. Contraceptively, it is difficult to block millions of sperm, easier to focus on one ovum.

Nevertheless, the two contraceptive methods available to males are among the most effective and trouble-free. The condom has particular advantages in that it is the only contraceptive method that also provides protection against STDs/HIV. In fact, since greater awareness of safer sex, condom use has dramatically increased. Having a condom readily available is a symbol of male awareness and responsibility. For a single man or man engaged in extramarital relationships, protection against STDs/HIV is crucial, particularly if he has several partners. Condoms are available in drugstores and grocery stores where they can be purchased unobtrusively. It is also possible to purchase condoms through the mail. Condoms do not require a doctor's visit or prescription, and are relatively inexpensive. The quality of condoms has improved markedly in recent years so they interfere less with penile sensations. Condoms are available lubricated and nonlubricated, in different colors, with deluxe features such as a receptacle at the tip to hold the ejaculate. Although available in lamb or natural membrane, latex condoms are much superior in protecting against STDs/HIV. Contrary to popular belief few condoms are defective (provided you do not buy bargain brands), so there is no need to test them by blowing air into them or filling them with water. Don't pretest or unwrap a condom, it's likely to cause damage. Use a condom only once, to reuse is penny-wise and pound foolish (an unwanted pregnancy). The condom is one of the few contraceptive methods free of side effects.

To be effective, the condom must be used in an optimal manner. Even among regular condom users only 60 percent use them optimally. A condom should not be put on until just before intercourse when the penis is erect. Some men enter the woman without the condom, then withdraw and place it on their penis when they are ready to ejaculate—an extremely risky technique we strongly recommend against. Even if the man is sure of his ability to control ejaculation, there is considerable risk because well before ejaculation there is a discharge from the Cowper's glands that contains enough live sperm to cause conception. This is why coitus interruptus is an unreliable contraceptive technique, even if the male withdraws well before ejaculation.

The condom should be put on so there is a half-inch space at the tip to accommodate the ejaculated semen (some condoms are made with a receptacle). Immediately after ejaculation, the penis should be withdrawn from the vagina. While withdrawing, it is critical that you hold the base of the condom to prevent spillage of the ejaculate into the vagina. This is the most violated guideline. Withdrawing right after ejaculation disrupts the lovemaking process. Often she urges him to stay close and connected. Although this is a healthy psychological need, it's an unhealthy and unnecessary risk in terms of pregnancy (as well as STDs/HIV). Our suggestion is to immediately withdraw, throw the condom in the trash basket (wipe off if you want) and come back to bed for afterplay or cuddling.

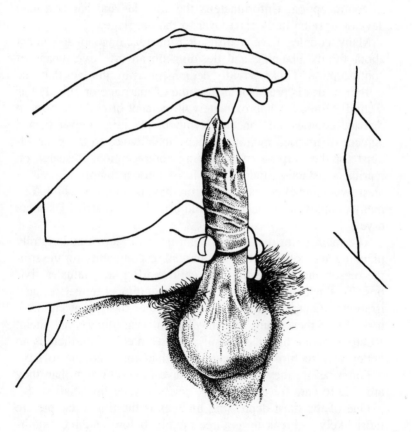

The woman putting on her partner's condom before intercourse.
Care is taken to allow about half-an-inch of space at the top to
accommodate ejaculated semen.

MARRIED MEN AND CONTRACEPTION

We have focused primarily on the use of contraceptives among single men. The rationale is that it is among single men that self-defeating attitudes and misconceptions are most prevalent. Married men do not share these uncaring and irresponsible attitudes, if only because they cannot afford to. Because a man is legally and financially responsible for children, he must take an interest in contraception. Unfortunately, the attitudes and habits a man develops premaritally carry over to the marriage.

Many couples have a difficult time reaching an agreement about family planning and deciding on an effective means of contraception. This is vividly demonstrated by the fact that one in four brides is pregnant at the time of marriage or already has a child. Moreover, approximately 40 percent of children born to married couples are conceived without planning. Fewer than 5 percent of married men accompany their wives to the gynecologist for the purpose of discussing contraception. Research on marital satisfaction indicates it is best for a couple to wait at least two years after marriage before having their first child. Yet, many couples have their first child after being married less than a year.

The main point that we, as men, need to recognize is family planning and contraception is a mutual responsibility for the simple reason that procreation and child rearing are mutual activities. To duck our share of the responsibility is unrealistic and irrational. Couples should discuss whether they want children, how many they want, and at what intervals they want them. "Letting nature take its course" may seem easy, but, there is no better way to turn a marriage sour than for a couple to have children before they are ready or have more children than they are able to care for emotionally, practically, or financially.

One of the most depressing findings is the time a couple are most likely to break up is three months before or three months after the birth of a first child. The couple needs to be sure their marriage is viable before having a planned, wanted child and beginning the transition to a three person family. A child will not save a tenuous marriage, it's more likely to stress the couple and destroy the marital bond.

The couple needs to fully explore their thoughts, feelings and practical considerations regarding contraceptive methods. Both partners must realize there is not a "perfect" contraceptive. They need to be aware of the advantages as well as problems and side effects and choose a contraceptive which is comfortable and functional for them.

FEMALE CONTRACEPTIVES

There are two categories of female contraceptives, hormonal and barrier. The major hormonal methods are birth control pills, Depo-Provera injections, and Norplant. The major barrier methods are the IUD, diaphragm, cervical cap, and vaginal spermicides. The birth control pill—the most popular contraceptive— is the most effective. The woman takes the pill daily. The synthetic hormones (estrogen and progestin) in the pill prevent ovulation (the releasing of the egg), therefore pregnancy cannot occur even though she continues to have a regular menstrual period. It is crucial to undergo periodic examinations (usually once a year) with her gynecologist because a minority of women have disturbing or serious side effects including headaches, blood clots, high blood pressure, depression, and inhibited sexual desire. For the majority, the birth control pill is a safe and effective means of contraception. It has the important advantage of separating sexual expression and contraception.

Depo-Provera injections (typically given every three months) are preferred by women who find taking a pill daily is difficult. Although convenient, many women find side effects, especially nausea and breakthrough bleeding (small amounts of menstrual blood), hard to adapt to.

Norplant surgical implants have the major benefit of contraceptive protection for up to five years after the gynecologist inserts them. Although cheaper in the long run, it is a major upfront financial expense as well as a commitment to not have children for a number of years. Some women complain of weight gain and have a difficult time adjusting to alterations in their menstrual flow.

The intrauterine device (IUD), which ranks second only to the pill in effectiveness, is a copper loop placed in the uterus by a gynecologist. Once in position, it remains there until there is a reason to take it out (for example, if the couple desire a pregnancy) or after three years. The IUD must be removed by a physician. One advantage of the IUD is it does not entail a daily routine, as does the pill, or application before each sexual encounter, as do the diaphragm and condom. The strings of the IUD should be checked monthly to make sure the device has not been spontaneously expelled. Although it is uncertain exactly how the IUD works, it does prevent implantation of the egg in the uterus. Some women experience unpleasant side effects such as irregular bleeding. The biggest dangers with the IUD are it can perforate the uterine wall, cause infection, or be spontaneously expelled. The woman needs to be sure her gynecologist is expert at IUD insertion. IUDs were difficult to obtain for a time, as manufacturers removed them from the market because of liability lawsuits. IUDs have recently regained popularity, particularly among women who've had a child.

A dome-shaped, thin rubber cup stretched over a flexible ring, the diaphragm is designed to cover the entrance to the cervix. It's inserted into the vagina prior to intercourse. A spermicidal cream or jelly, which is toxic for sperm, is placed on the rubber dome and around the rim of the diaphragm. When used properly, the diaphragm is a safe and highly effective contraceptive. Insert it not more than two hours before intercourse for optimal effectiveness. If you are going to have intercourse a second time, another application of jelly or cream must be used via a special insertion device. The woman must keep the diaphragm in place for at least six hours after intercourse. The most common complaint about the diaphragm is it interferes with sexual spontaneity. The diaphragm has made a comeback in popularity because of its lack of side effects. Some couples make putting in the diaphragm a part of foreplay/pleasuring. Use of the condom and diaphragm together is extremely effective in preventing pregnancy and STDs/HIV. The major difficulty with the diaphragm is motivation for use each time—many couples become lazy, are swept away by the passion of the moment, or feel they can risk it "just this once." Women who are regularly orgasmic during intercourse, especially when using the woman on top position, are at greater risk for conception because the diaphragm can temporarily move away from the cervix. The practical failure rate of the diaphragm is higher than its theoretical failure rate (similar to condoms and other barrier methods). Women who gain or lose ten pounds, who have had a child or abortion, or who report discomfort after use should consult the gynecologist to reevaluate diaphragm fit. Rigorous, optimal utilization is required for diaphragm effectiveness.

Some women prefer the cervical cap to the diaphragm. The cervical cap is like a miniature diaphragm, it fits over the cervix and can be left in place for up to 24 hours. The woman has to weigh the pros and cons of the cap compared to the diaphragm. Other forms of female birth control include foams and spermicides. These are only moderately effective, and are not recommended unless used with a condom.

Since the most popular and effective forms of female contraception require a gynecological exam and prescription, the next step is to consult a gynecologist. We encourage the man to accompany his partner to the appointment and share in discussion of the alternatives. If this is not possible, discuss her visit afterward and offer support for the contraceptive method she chose. He should not delude himself into thinking she alone is responsible. Each couple has to choose a form of contraception that is comfortable for them and can be used in a conscientious, effective manner.

If a couple has decided to use the pill, the man should adopt the attitude that, if she skips a day, it is *they* who have forgotten to take *their* pill. The same is true for use of the IUD and diaphragm. Instead of the woman inserting the diaphragm by herself in private, the man should ask if the diaphragm is in or continues to hold and caress her as she does the insertion. If she uses an IUD, he should make a habit of checking the string monthly to be sure it remains in place. Responsibility for advising the woman on what kind of birth control pill to use or fitting a diaphragm falls on the gynecologist, but the man can take an intelligent part in the discussion, decision, and implementation. Working together on contraception can enhance feelings of mutuality in all aspects of the relationship.

Recently, there has been a great deal of publicity about the female pouch (female condom). This appeals to women who want to feel responsible in protecting against STDs/HIV. Since it is more expensive and awkward than the male condom and appears to be a less effective contraceptive, we suggest couples use the male condom and/or another form of birth control.

When contraception has failed—religious and moral questions

aside—abortion is a viable, though not ideal, alternative. Abortion is an expensive, minor surgical procedure, and it can trigger difficult psychological reactions. Ideally, abortions should be done on an outpatient basis at a clinic under a local anesthetic. Legally, in the U.S., abortions of this type must be performed within three months of conception. When an unwanted pregnancy occurs, and the man and woman decide abortion is the best solution, the man should support his partner both financially and emotionally. The same principles apply here as with contraceptive techniques.

CONTRACEPTION AS AN ONGOING PROCESS

The question of contraception is not settled forever after the initial visit to the gynecologist. Although many contraceptive methods are effective, there is no perfect contraceptive. Contraceptive devices are judged according to several criteria: reliability, convenience, interference with sexual pleasure, freedom from side effects, expense, and, finally, the ease with which it is reversible. A woman is fertile until menopause, and a man is fertile into his sixties and beyond. Couples need to periodically discuss and reevaluate the contraceptive method they are using to ensure it continues to suit their needs.

STERILIZATION

The most popular form of birth control for people over 35 are tubal ligation and vasectomy. There are two major reasons for this: first, one or both people have decided they want no more children and second, after years of switching methods and fearing pregnancy, they are tired of the hassles of contraception. Sterilization is reliable, convenient, doesn't interfere with sexual pleasure, has few or no side effects, and is relatively inexpensive. What it isn't is easily reversible. Sterilization is best thought of as a permanent decision (closing the chapter on childbearing).

Let us first examine the male form of sterilization, vasectomy.

MISCONCEPTIONS ABOUT VASECTOMY

Sterilization suffers, unfortunately, from negative connotations. Sterilization has been used as a coercive measure to prevent individuals judged to be socially undesirable, such as criminals or mentally retarded people, from reproducing. Hence, it is thought of as punitive in nature.

Another negative is the confusion between vasectomy and castration. Even though a man might understand intellectually that the two operations are totally different, he retains an emotional aversion for anything that bears even a superficial resemblance to the "loss of manhood." The fact castration is used as a means of sterilizing pets and farm animals adds unpleasant connotations. Men tend to balk at any situation involving the close proximity of their testicles and a sharp instrument.

Vasectomy has nothing in common with castration, either in the mechanics of the operation or its aftereffects. Castration involves the removal of the testicles. Vasectomy, on the other hand, is a simple and safe minor surgical procedure in which the vas deferens, two small tubes leading from the testicles, are cut and tied so the sperm does not proceed to the penis. The testicles continue to produce sperm, but it is absorbed into the body rather than becoming part of the ejaculate. The total volume and force of ejaculation does not diminish. Ninety-seven percent of the ejaculate is composed of semen, which is not affected by the vasectomy. The sensations accompanying ejaculation do not change, and there is no loss of pleasure. Nor is there a change in the capacity to experience desire or have erections.

Sexual desire is regulated in part by testosterone, a hormone produced in the testicles which enters the body through the bloodstream. Testosterone is unaffected by sterilization. It is extremely unusual for a male to develop desire or erection problems after a vasectomy. In cases where a sexual problem develops, the cause is almost always psychological or relational rather than physical. In fact, sexual desire usually increases after vasectomy for both partners because sexuality is no longer inhibited by fear of pregnancy. To repeat, the only effect of a vasectomy is to eliminate the male's ability to have children; there are no changes in desire, erection, or orgasm.

THE VASECTOMY PROCEDURE

There are some common misconceptions about vasectomy—some think it is a lengthy and expensive procedure, requires a general anesthetic, requires a hospital stay, involves painful aftereffects, and requires time for convalescence. Men are amazed that an operation with such a profound effect on their lives entails less pain and discomfort than a visit to the dentist. Vasectomy is a minor surgical procedure performed in the urologist's office. The operation takes about fifteen minutes, and the total time spent in the office is less than an hour. The majority of vasectomy operations are performed by private urologists, with the cost sometimes covered by medical insurance. Many cities have outpatient vasectomy clinics attached to a medical center where the operation is offered at a lower fee.

After administering a local anesthetic, the urologist makes two small incisions in the scrotum and cuts and ties the vas deferens. The potential for side effects and complications is minimal.

Vasectomy involves little or no discomfort or interruption in the man's activities. There may be soreness lasting for one to three days after the surgery. During this time, the male is advised to refrain from strenuous activity, and may want to wear an athletic supporter. There should be no reason for him to miss more than one day of work, if even that. Usually there is a small swelling on each testicle, but this disappears in a week.

USE OF CONTRACEPTION AFTER VASECTOMY

The man does not become sterile immediately after the operation. Sperm remain in the upper part of the vas, in the seminal vesicles, and in the ejaculatory ducts, so ten to sixteen ejaculations are required to "clean out" the sperm from the semen. During this time, contraception must be used. Contraception should not be dispensed with until after the patient is checked to make sure his semen contains no sperm. For this test, the man can have intercourse using a condom, masturbate, or have his partner stimulate him to orgasm and collect the ejaculate in a jar. He brings the sample to the laboratory for analysis. A similar examination should be conducted six months later to make sure the vas has not grown back together. This is an extremely rare occurrence, but the second test is an important precaution.

REVERSIBILITY

The question most often raised is the possibility of a "reversible vasectomy." Although there are microsurgery techniques to rejoin the vas and pregnancies occur (especially in men who reverse the vasectomy in less than five years), vasectomy should be considered a permanent procedure. The structural restoration of the vas does not guarantee renewed fertility. A technique that had been researched was a spigot that could be implanted in the vas and used to start and stop the flow of sperm. However, along with the technical difficulties of perfecting the spigot, there is an added problem—when the sperm are not being used, there is a decrease in sperm production and the viability of the sperm produced. The sperm might no longer be effective, and a man would have difficulty impregnating his wife.

One possible way of dealing with the irreversibility issue is to deposit sperm in a sperm bank, where it is frozen and stored, prior to having a vasectomy. If the couple later decided to have more children, the husband's sperm could be used to inseminate her artificially. However, one cannot be assured of success.

Another procedure is use of donor sperm. This is a commonly used and accepted procedure in the treatment of infertility. The husband and wife are advised to examine their attitudes and feelings carefully before choosing insemination by donor sperm. In addition to discussing technical aspects of donor insemination with the fertility specialist, we suggest you discuss psychological issues with a mental health clinician who has a subspecialty in infertility.

ADVANTAGES

The irreversibility of the vasectomy is its only major drawback. According to the other criteria by which we judge the worth of contraceptive methods, vasectomy rates extremely high.

For couples who have completed their childbearing, the husband's decision to have a vasectomy can rejuvenate their sexual relationship. Alan, a thirty-eight-year-old client of Barry's, married sixteen years and the father of three children, is a case in point. Two of Alan's children had been unplanned, and the problem of contraception was a major inhibiting factor in their sexual relationship. They had tried almost everything and were now using a condom along with spermicidal foam. Sex could not really be spontaneous under these conditions. Alan had not thought of a vasectomy until a friend had one. At first he was reluctant even to discuss it because of fears the operation would make him less masculine or less sexual. His attitude improved when he read literature about vasectomy and learned the facts from his internist. Alan had a consultation (to which his wife accompanied him) with the urologist. After much thought and several discussions with his wife, Alan decided vasectomy would be the best choice. He felt anxious on the day of the operation, but found to his surprise it was "easier than having a tooth pulled." There were no complications. Alan and his wife enjoyed spontaneous sex, free of contraceptive concerns. Intercourse frequency and satisfaction increased to a level they had not experienced since the birth of their first child.

PERSONAL EXPERIENCE

Like Alan, the majority of men find a vasectomy has a positive effect on their sexual relationship and lives in general. One of the most difficult elements in Barry's decision to have a vasectomy was he had been very involved in Emily's two pregnancies and thoroughly enjoyed the process of having and parenting children. A vasectomy meant giving up the possibility of having another child. However, we decided two biological children and one adopted child were enough. Being voluntarily sterile has given our sexual relationship greater freedom. Barry has no regrets.

CANDIDATES FOR VASECTOMY

A couple should frankly and maturely discuss the issues involved, and only when they are satisfied vasectomy is the best answer to their family planning needs should the man have the operation. Vasectomy is not for everyone. It would not be a wise choice for a young, unmarried man or a couple who are uncertain whether they want more children. Nor would it be a good choice for the man who is divorced or contemplating divorce and may wish to have children with a new spouse.

For a man who has decided, along with his wife, that he has

as many children as he wants and wishes to be free of the possibility of an unwanted pregnancy, it is the ideal alternative. Single, widowed, or divorced men who are certain they wish to father no more children are excellent candidates for vasectomy. Each year, approximately 100,000 vasectomies are performed in the United States. Vasectomy is gaining in popularity in other parts of the world as well.

The fact vasectomy is a male-oriented contraceptive method, that it allows the man to take the initiative, is very much in its favor. Male sterilization allows us to assume responsibility for family planning. This is a major contribution toward establishing the atmosphere of trust which is essential to a vital sexual relationship. When done in a spirit of understanding and cooperation, a vasectomy serves to show how much he cares about his wife and his commitment to their marriage. Of course, if there are serious problems in the marriage, it is unlikely a vasectomy will resolve them. But if the relationship is good, the husband's decision can and often does improve the marriage by providing greater trust and sexual freedom.

TUBAL LIGATION

There are approximately three times as many women who obtain tubal ligations as men who have vasectomies. This was true even when tubal ligations were a major surgical procedure, done under general anesthesia, expensive, and medically risky. Happily, the technology of tubal ligation has dramatically improved in the past decade. Tubal ligation is now done on an outpatient basis, with a local anesthetic, is less expensive, and low risk. Still, from a medical viewpoint, vasectomy is the preferred procedure. Then why are there more tubal ligations than vasectomies?

DECIDING WHICH PARTNER SHOULD BE
STERILIZED

Sterilization is best made as a joint decision. There are cases in which female sterilization would be the best alternative—if, for example, the man had an aversion to vasectomy, while the woman felt strongly committed to sterilization. A thorough discussion by the couple, as well as a consultation with a gynecologist, should precede surgery.

The decision should be based on two factors. First, which spouse is more committed to not having another child? It is usually the more motivated person who opts for the sterilization procedure. Often, this is the woman. The second factor involves psychological and sexual comfort. One partner might be anxious about surgery. Sexually oriented surgery might have a bigger impact on the self-image or sexual confidence of one partner. For example, the woman might attach major significance to reproduction as the core of her femininity and sexual desirability. The man might become sexually self-conscious or anxious after a vasectomy. The partner who has a stable sense of body image and sexuality is the one who volunteers for sterilization.

No man should allow himself to be pressured into having a vasectomy. If he feels ambivalent about the procedure, it would be best not to proceed. His decision should be based on his true feelings. The most undesirable consequence of a vasectomy would be for the man to be sorry or angry and feel he'd been victimized.

VASECTOMY AS A POSITIVE CHOICE

The choice of a vasectomy should be made freely, with the man understanding the operation and its effects. He should feel comfortable with his masculinity and sexuality both before and after the operation. Sterility is an unfortunate condition only for men who want to father children. When parenthood is no longer desired, sterility becomes a positive good because it gives the man freedom to express himself sexually without fear of an unwanted pregnancy. Sterilization is the primary choice of contraception for couples after their mid-thirties.

4

SEXUAL HEALTH—STDS AND HIV

STDs, sexually transmitted diseases, present the depressing reality that you can get a disease from making love. HIV (Human Immunodeficiency Virus) causes AIDS (Autoimmune Deficiency Syndrome) so you can die from making love. STDs and HIV/ AIDS, a potential consequence of sex, are a very serious health concern. Awareness of sexual risk is literally a matter of life and death.

With the worldwide fears of HIV/AIDS, people have largely ignored the much more common STDs. HIV is an STD, although it can also be transmitted by blood, i.e., through use of contaminated needles. AIDS is fatal where STDs seldom are. However, psychologically and medically, ignoring STDs is a mistake. If you are aware and committed to protecting your sexual health, you need to be aware of ''safer sex'' strategies which will protect you from a range of diseases, not just HIV. You want to conduct your sexual life so it adds to your physical and emotional well-being, and does not become a source of fear or illness.

It is important to keep one distinction firmly in mind. You don't get an STD (or HIV) *because* you have sex. It isn't a judgment, a punishment, a bacterial sword of Damocles waiting to fall on the sexual transgressor. You contract an STD through sex contact, which is very different. The idea that an STD is a penalty for sex has long been used by moralists for the suppression of sexual activity. It is an old and tenacious fallacy, akin to the notion that plagues came about as a direct result of sinful behavior. There has been a resurgence of this type of thinking because of AIDS, herpes, and genital warts—three STDs that are not curable. That such ideas still garner acceptance attests to the capacity of human beings to feel guilt and shame. The medieval plagues were caused not by sin but by poor sanitation. Similarly, the current epidemic of STDs is not a punishment for increased sexuality, but the result of ignorance and lack of sexual responsibility. It is the consequence of our failure to face a problem squarely, to plan our sexual activities, and to take responsibility for our sexual health.

Avoiding sex because it can give you an STD is not the answer. After all, you can contract influenza by breathing in viruses and can catch hepatitis by eating contaminated food—hardly valid reasons for avoiding the company of others or refusing to eat. The answer is not to avoid sex, but be aware of how to prevent, detect, and treat STDs so this medical problem does not interfere with your life and sexuality.

DATA ABOUT STDS

Connected with the idea that STDs are a punishment for sexual activity is the notion that only morally "degenerate" or "dirty" people contract STDs. Men believe an STD "can't happen to me," it is contracted only by a group of people who are inferior to oneself. When a man contracts an STD, his reaction is one of intense surprise and shame: "This can't be happening to me—not me!" He feels having an STD brands him as a socially and morally undesirable individual. He turns on the sex partner he suspects of giving him the STD and accuses her of being a "whore." This attitude makes little sense when one considers the extreme prevalence of STDs. In 1996, 5 million Americans contracted an STD. It is estimated that in their lifetime 40 percent of Americans will contract at least one STD. In the face of such numbers, it becomes clear STDs must be taken seriously by all of us.

The group most at risk for STDs is the young. The highest incidence rate is among individuals between the ages of fifteen and nineteen. But STDs attack people of all ages, races, religions, sexual orientations, and socioeconomic groups. If you think for a moment about the extent of the networks formed in our society through sexual contact, it becomes obvious there are few people who are not potential STD victims. An STD is a medical disease, not a moral judgment.

How does one contract an STD? And what are the most common? The five most common STDs are chlamydia, herpes, genital warts, gonorrhea, and syphilis. HIV/AIDS is not among the most common STDs, although it is the most lethal. Heterosexual intercourse is not the only way STDs are transmitted. STDs are contracted through oral and anal sex. They can be transmitted through homosexual as well as heterosexual contacts. In fact, the STD rate among homosexual males is considerably higher than among heterosexual males.

Chlamydia (in males it's also called nongonococcal urethritis—NGU) is the most common STD in the U.S. Each year approximately 3 million people contract chlamydia. It is an organism spread by sexual contact that infects the genitals of males and females. In males, the symptoms are a thin, clear discharge and mild pain on urination. Females are usually asymptomatic. One of the reasons for its high level is that partners reinfect one another. It is essential both partners be treated at the same time and they cease being sexual until cured.

Herpes can only be diagnosed when there is an active outbreak of sores. When this occurs go to your internist, urologist, or dermatologist who will take a scraping from the sores, analyze it, and tell you whether it is herpes. If you have herpes, you need to be an aware patient but not overreact. There is no cure for herpes, but its effects are less severe than for other STDs. Some people will have a single herpes outbreak, then the disease will remain dormant. A typical pattern is for herpes outbreaks to start weeks apart, and gradually decrease in frequency and intensity. It is crucial for the man to be aware of his herpes cycle and refrain from any contact with the herpes sores during an outbreak (or during your partner's outbreak). Even if both people already have herpes, abstinence from sexual contact should be rigidly adhered to because of reinfection by additional herpes viruses. During a herpes outbreak, the infected person can stimulate the partner, but great care must be taken to avoid all contact with herpes sores.

Genital warts are the most increasing category of STDs. Unfortunately, unlike gonorrhea, chlamydia and syphilis, genital warts is in the same category as herpes—a chronic infection which can be monitored and treated, but not cured. There are 65 types of genital warts. It is important to be aware of and treat genital warts and avoid partner sexual contact until the warts are gone. In many ways, genital warts are similar to herpes.

Gonorrhea is passed from person to person by genital contact (penis-vagina, oral-genital, or anal intercourse). Major symptoms are a burning sensation during urination and a heavy discharge of whitish or yellowish pus from the penis, while typically, women are asymptomatic. At least the man realizes he has an STD and needs to be treated (the woman is dependent on him to tell her she's infected and must seek treatment). Treatment requires specific medication with a follow-up genital culture to ensure the infection is eradicated.

Syphilis is transmitted by close, intimate contact that is usually, but not always, sexual. It is possible for syphilis to be transmitted by kissing if one of the partners has a chancre in his mouth. The germs that cause syphilis die very quickly if they are not in a warm, moist environment. Thus, contrary to popular notions, it is impossible to catch syphilis through contact with unsanitary toilet seats or from towels. Untreated syphilis can result in organ damage and even death. The disappearance of symptoms does not mean the disease is gone, it is infecting the body internally. Treatment is crucial.

Other STDs include trichomoniasis, pubic lice (crabs), and chancroid. Consult a physician if you have any reason to fear you have contracted an STD. Ask to have a full check for the range of STDs, and be sure to fully comply with the treatment program.

HIV/AIDS

The terms HIV (Human Immunodeficiency Virus) and AIDS (Acquired Immune Deficiency Syndrome) are enough to cause terror in men and women throughout the world. AIDS is a new disease, not diagnosed until 1980. AIDS is a serious public health threat and has become a worldwide epidemic. However, the atmosphere of fear, stigma, and moralistic pandering to people's misconceptions by calling it God's revenge on homosexuals, nature's way of containing sex, or God's punishment for sexual wickedness, is untrue and counterproductive.

Let us examine the presently known scientific facts about AIDS from an objective standpoint and discuss how we can be responsible, practice safer sex, and guard our sexual health.

First, HIV is a virus that is spread primarily through the mediums of blood and semen. Vaginal secretions can spread HIV, but it's a much less powerful medium. Although present in other mediums—saliva, tears, sweat—it is very unlikely the disease will be transmitted that way. The only good news about the HIV virus is that it is difficult to transmit. Fortunately, saliva, tears, and sweat do not contain enough concentration of the virus to infect another person.

Second, HIV/AIDS is not a disease of sexual orientation; it can be transmitted to both heterosexuals and homosexuals. In some countries, AIDS is more common among heterosexuals than homosexuals.

Third, when it comes to sexual contact (as opposed to blood transmission) HIV/AIDS is a disease passed from males to females or males to males. Transmission from female to male, although possible, is less frequent. It is fifteen times easier to transmit HIV male to female than female to male. A male who has the HIV virus infects a female by semen entering her vagina, anus, and to a lesser degree through fellatio.

Fourth, the carriers of HIV/AIDS are healthy men who have no symptoms, but once infected are always contagious and are carriers indefinitely.

Fifth, the means of transmission sexually is through semen entering the other person's body whether through vaginal or anal transmission, and to a lesser extent oral-genital transmission.

The reason there have been so many cases of AIDS in the homosexual community is the number of sexual partners some gay men have (thus, the carrier infects many men) and the use of anal intercourse (which can break small blood vessels in the anal area, thus mixing blood and semen, which presents the greatest risk for HIV transmission). People who are passive in anal intercourse are the highest risk group for HIV/AIDS.

PREVENTION OF HIV/AIDS

Since at present there is no cure for AIDS and it is a terminal disease, prevention is the obvious answer. Rather than talking about "safe sex" as a perfect guarantee, it is more reasonable to talk about "safer sex" strategies and techniques. Sexually (as opposed to through blood or needles), HIV is considerably easier to transmit by males (whether through heterosexual or homosexual contact) because alkaline semen is a more efficient medium for the virus than acid vaginal secretions. Vaginal and anal intercourse are far more dangerous for the woman than the man. In other words, the transmission is most often from man to woman or man to man. Female-to-male transmission is quite difficult. The exception is childbirth: women can transmit HIV to their babies and through breast milk.

One of the scariest aspects of the epidemic is HIV carriers are healthy people who have no symptoms and are usually unaware they are HIV positive. Once infected, the victim stays contagious, even though not ill. People with HIV eventually become ill with AIDS, but not for several years (the average is five to ten years).

There are three levels of prevention for men. The first is to limit your sexual activity to heterosexual sex, not do drugs with needles, and not have sex with prostitutes. For the woman it is to limit her sexual activity to partners who only function heterosexually, don't go to prostitutes, and do not use intravenous drugs.

The second level is to be sure the person you are sexual with is HIV negative. You need to have a direct, assertive conversation about STDs and HIV, to determine if the person is at risk. If you establish an ongoing relationship, you should assertively request both of you be tested for HIV (and STDs). Clinics and some private doctors allow you to take the test using a number or fictitious name (to ensure confidentiality) and to pay cash (so the transaction would not be recorded for health insurance purposes). Many clinics offer free and confidential testing for HIV. HIV screening tests are reliable and valid. You should be retested six months after your last risky sexual experience.

The third level of prevention is to practice safer sex. This means not allowing a person to ejaculate inside of you (anally or orally, and for women vaginally). The major safer sex procedure is for the male to wear a condom in vaginal, oral, and anal sex. If you are unsure of the HIV status of your partner, it is strongly recommended you use a condom each time.

SAFER SEX FOR SINGLE MEN

How can someone who is not in a monogamous relationship practice safer sex? The more aware, knowledgeable, and responsible you are about sexuality, the more you can protect your health against HIV/AIDS and other STDs.

Like other STDs, HIV has a "sexist" bias. It is much easier to transfer the HIV virus from males to females than from females to males. With gonorrhea, 90 percent of men are symptomatic, while less than 25 percent of women are, therefore the woman is dependent on the male to be honest and tell her that she needs to be tested and treated. She needs to be assertive in asking her partner whether he is "at risk" in terms of homosexual activity, IV drug use, or being sexual with prostitutes (the highest risk groups for HIV infection), keeping in mind that it is sexual behavior—not types of people—which spreads the HIV virus.

The best method is for both to be tested for HIV and other STDs and have an agreement to not be sexual with others—which means you have to trust your partner to be honest if there is an incident. The second-best preventive is to avoid activities involving exchange of semen and/or vaginal secretions. The highest risk activity is anal intercourse, followed by vaginal intercourse. Oral sex is less risky, especially if the male does not ejaculate into the woman's mouth. Many couples use condoms during fellatio or a dental dam during cunnilingus. If you are unsure of the partner's health status, always use condoms.

HIV/AIDS is a very serious problem that needs to be addressed by both men and women, heterosexuals and homosexuals. The better informed you are, the more you can objectively determine how to behave in a safer-sex, health-promoting manner. People governed by fears and panic do not take beneficial steps; people who value themselves and their sexuality will do what is necessary to protect their health.

IF A PERSON TESTS POSITIVE

A positive result on the HIV screening test means you have the HIV antibodies in your bloodstream and will be a carrier (contagious) all your life. You can protect your immune system by living an especially healthy life. This means good eating, sleeping, and exercising habits, not smoking or using drugs, and moderate drinking. Immediately consult a physician with a sub-specialty practice in HIV/AIDS about preventative medication and steps you can take to protect your health and immune system.

A positive HIV test means a dramatic change in your sexual behavior. You will not be able to engage in any sexual activity that involves exchange of body fluids, that is, you cannot ejaculate inside anyone or have them ejaculate inside you. You can engage in sensual and sexual expression, but it needs to be limited; you can stimulate yourself or your partner can manually stimulate you to orgasm, but don't utilize oral sex, anal sex, or vaginal intercourse. We strongly urge you to join a support group with other HIV positive people. The group can provide emotional encouragement as well as correct information and practical suggestions.

With increased medical research and drug interventions, it's likely AIDS will become a manageable chronic medical condition, like diabetes and multiple sclerosis. The first level of management is maintaining good health, protecting your immune system, and maintaining your T-cell count above 200. Increasingly, physicians are urging men to be regularly tested for HIV, and if they are positive to immediately begin taking medication which combats the development of the virus.

PREVENTION OF STDS

Sexual comfort requires sexual health and safer sex. The safest sex involves a couple who are intimate, committed, and free of STDs. This allows the full range of sexual experiences and provides freedom from fear of disease. Is that too idealistic? A new tradition among committed or married couples is to be tested for HIV and other STDs. You agree to inform the partner if either engages in any risky sexual activity with another person. If so, the couple will have a full check for the range of STDs, then a condom will be used until the couple is retested for HIV six months later. This involves trust in yourself and your partner to be responsible and honor the agreement.

When Barry first began teaching a college sexuality course in 1970, the major STDs were gonorrhea and syphilis. In the 1970s, herpes began to spread and became the most feared STD because it has no cure. Herpes was and is a serious STD which affects over 20 million Americans, but its effects can be dealt with and are less devastating than originally feared. The most frequently contracted STD is chlamydia, which results in 3 million new cases each year. However, with the furor over HIV/AIDS, STDs have been forgotten (which is not wise). HIV/AIDS has dominated sexuality since the 1980s and will probably do so for the foreseeable future, yet it is not among the most common STDs.

STDs are not irrational fears. During their lifetime, approximately four in ten people will contract an STD. STDs need to be dealt with as a health problem, not a moral judgment. The atmosphere of fear and stigma is counterproductive, as well as untrue.

DEALING WITH AN STD RATIONALLY

An STD, because of its peculiar symptomatology, can be difficult to detect (especially for women) and often goes untreated. However, the medical difficulties of treating the disease are insignificant compared with the psychological resistance that prevents its victims from dealing with an STD in a rational manner. Particular diseases affect our images of people in particular ways. Certain diseases are socially acceptable, others are not. A man who has suffered a heart attack may feel despondent that his body has failed him, but not hide the nature of his disease. However, people feel intense shame when they find they are suffering from an STD. They feel the disease identifies them with the world of prostitutes, of seamy, lower-class characters suffering the consequences of sexual excesses. So intense is this shame that many victims will not allow themselves to believe they actually have an STD, even after the symptoms manifest themselves unmistakably.

People who contract STDs avoid obtaining treatment or wait so long before seeing a doctor that complications occur which lead to permanent damage. Other victims seek treatment, but go to great lengths to "hush it up." Unfortunately, many doctors are willing to cater to this anxiety. STD cases are supposed to be reported to the health department. The information about sexual partners, embarrassing as it may be to divulge, is necessary so those who have been exposed can be notified, tested, and treated. Symptoms are not always noticeable, especially among women, so they are unaware they have an STD. Meanwhile, the infection may spread from one person to another until dozens, perhaps hundreds, have been affected.

The microorganisms that cause STDs have no interest in the social status of their victims. As far as STDs are concerned, we are all one big family. It makes no more sense to be ashamed of catching an STD than it does to be ashamed of catching the flu. Moreover, whatever shame may be connected with an STD should be more than outweighed by a sense of responsibility to your well-being, to society in general, and especially to the people you choose as sex partners. Responsibility ought to be the keynote of all our sexual involvements.

In view of the ease with which most STDs can be cured, there is no excuse for them to have grown to epidemic proportions. Public information and advertising campaigns aim at providing accurate information concerning STDs. Free STD clinics treat patients confidentially, including those under legal age.

Despite these efforts, the incidence of STDs is still on the increase. The shame connected with the disease continues. Until steps are taken to correct this situation, irrational and self-defeating behavior will remain the rule. The public's attitude toward STDs resembles the syndrome of fear, denial, and embarrassment that surrounded breast cancer and prevented women from being tested and seeking treatment. The turning point occurred in the 1970s, when, in rapid succession, Betty Ford and Happy Rockefeller announced they had breast cancer. The example set by these two public figures—the wives of the president and vice president—encouraged women to learn about breast cancer, do monthly breast self-exams, and obtain yearly examinations by a gynecologist. As a result, there has been a dramatic increase in the detection of breast cancer in its early stages. It would be a great step toward bringing STDs and HIV under control if public figures were to perform a similar service with respect to these diseases. Considering their prevalence, there should not be a lack of opportunity. The example of courageous people, similar to Magic Johnson's disclosure of being HIV positive, would bring a much needed change in the public's attitude toward STDs, including HIV/AIDS.

MALE RESPONSIBILITY TO INFORM PARTNERS

In a sense, men are fortunate because the symptoms of STDs are distinct. The chances of detecting them in the early stages are much greater than in women, who usually have no symptoms. Reservations about seeking treatment are overcome by the obvious physical discomfort when a man who has gonorrhea or chlamydia experiences pain on urination or a discharge from his penis. Herpes sores and genital warts are more easily observed in males. The responsible and compassionate thing for the man to do if he has an STD is to inform anyone with whom he has had sexual contact. By doing so, he helps his partner detect an STD in its early stages and avoid the consequences of the later forms of the disease. The effects of untreated STDs are particularly severe in women and the danger is great that significant damage will occur before the disease is identified.

The problem of how to tell a partner she should be tested and, if necessary, treated for an STD is complex, particularly if informing her involves revealing you had sexual contacts she was unaware of. There is no "right" way to do this, but for the sake of your partner's health it is crucial to inform her. You can take the responsibility yourself or have medical authorities contact her. The latter alternative is the less courageous one, but it gets the job done, and that is the main thing. Whichever way you choose, and whatever the possible consequences to the relationship, the only sensible course of action is to tell your partner, since the health hazards of untreated STDs are so great.

Ralph

The discovery of an STD presents difficult psychological problems in addition to the obvious medical ones. Ralph, a twenty-eight-year-old salesman, was engaged to be married, but still indulged in casual affairs while on sales trips. Three months before the date for the wedding, during one such trip, he had sex with a woman he met in a bar. He came home on Friday and spent a sexually active weekend with his fiancée. Four days later, Ralph noticed a burning sensation during urination. Suspecting an STD, he went to his physician. The test results were positive for both gonorrhea and chlamydia, so the doctor treated Ralph, but did not urge him to supply the names of recent sex partners. Ralph had to decide what to tell his fiancée. For two days, he was tortured by doubts and indecision. He had no way of telling whether he had caught the STDs from the woman in the bar or his fiancée. If his fiancée was responsible, this meant she had another sex partner, and despite his own infidelities, Ralph found this infuriating. But whether she had infected him or not, chances were she had the disease and would have to be told. For several days Ralph attempted, through indirect questioning, to determine whether she'd had sex with another man. Finally, he told her. She accepted the news more calmly than he anticipated. Ralph went with her to the gynecologist for a smear and culture, which were positive. The episode was not pleasant for either of them, but she felt reassured about Ralph's concern for her welfare more than she felt hurt by his having sex with another woman. This was an impetus for them to make an agreement about affairs. Ralph committed to not having affairs, but if it occured he would use a condom and not have unprotected sex with his wife until he was tested. The wedding took place on schedule.

CLOSING THOUGHTS

Throughout this book it is assumed that the best and most realistic criterion for judging if a specific sexual practice is acceptable is whether it is harmful in some way to you or your partner. This includes vulnerability to HIV, STDs, unwanted pregnancy, physical pain, or psychological coercion. You cannot do yourself good by harming others. STDs and HIV greatly increase the possibility of harming others through sex or being harmed by them. STDs generally, and HIV/AIDS specifically, are "sexist" diseases; women are vulnerable to contracting it from male partners. Males are more likely to be aware of their STD status because they are symptomatic. This is not meant to promote hysteria or paranoia, but to make people aware that now more than ever it is crucial to establish respectful, trusting, and communicative relationships. The ethics governing one's attitude toward STDs and HIV are not different from the ethics of sexuality in general. Behavior that is based on awareness, caring, compassion, and responsibility will serve you well.

5

SELF-EXPLORATION AND MASTURBATION

The traditional manner used to discourage masturbation was fear and guilt—it was said to cause blindness, warts, poor sports performance, physical weakness, impotence, etc. Fathers warned sons to avoid "self-abuse" and threatened them with all kinds of punishments. Yet, the reality is 95 percent of males masturbate, most of them beginning between the ages of 10 and 14. Why? Because it's a normal, healthy part of male sexual development. While most boys and young men say masturbation feels good, few admit to an unabashed enthusiasm for it. Adolescents joke about masturbation and may at times masturbate either in pairs or groups. But once heterosexual relations become a reality, or even a possibility, masturbation is pushed into the closet. "I don't need it anymore," a young man says, which is a way of bragging his sex life is so full there is nothing left for autoeroticism. Seldom does such a boast come anywhere near the truth. The average young, unmarried male does not have intercourse frequently. Manual, oral, or rubbing stimulation to orgasm may account for another, somewhat larger, share of his sexual activity. The most frequent sexual outlet for adolescent and young adult men is masturbation; yet, it is only with reluctance and shame they admit this. Married men have an even tougher time confessing the truth. Surveys show a majority of men masturbate occasionally after marriage. Yet, most married men consider masturbation abnormal, an indulgence for which there is no justification.

Such an attitude is difficult to understand. Few of us believe masturbation is harmful. Nor would men deny it is pleasurable.

50

Is it not strange that an enhancing pleasure should generate such disapproval and guilt?

Actually, it is not strange at all when one considers the male machine attitude. Sex is a goal-oriented activity. The ultimate object is intercourse and orgasm; if the man "gives" his partner an orgasm, too, so much the better. Anything else is a failure or, perhaps, a mere step on the road to success. Adolescents will confront a peer returning from a date with the question "What did you get off her?" "I got tit" is pretty good. "I got two fingers in" is better. "She gave me a blow job" is a sign of triumph. But the greatest achievement is intercourse—to "score." The male who's scored the most frequently with the most partners is a source of envy. Where intercourse is concerned, particularly among young males, quantity is everything, quality practically nothing. The young man who reports he and his girlfriend caressed for an hour and it was a "fantastic experience" would be ridiculed by male friends.

Since intercourse is the male's goal, masturbation serves no practical purpose and is unjustified. All it produces is pleasure, and pleasure, from the traditional macho viewpoint, is not acceptable as a goal.

MASTURBATION AND GUILT

Because of the warnings we've been given about masturbation as children and because of its reputation as a poor sexual substitute, many of us feel guilty or at least self-conscious when we masturbate. This does not stop us from doing it, however. Embarrassment does prevent us from enjoying masturbation to the fullest and inhibits us from allowing masturbation to be the liberating and satisfying experience it can be. Most men are stubbornly goal-oriented in masturbation, to have an orgasm and relieve sexual tension. Consequently, we want to get done as quickly as possible—the sooner orgasm is reached, the better. We do not give ourselves the chance to realize masturbation, far from being a shameful necessity, is one of the best ways of learning about your sexual response cycle and increasing sensitivity to sexual stimulation—lessons that can be applied with enormous profit to partner sex.

It may come as a shock to hear masturbation recommended

so positively. We can almost hear a reader exclaiming, "You're actually telling guys it's good for them to jerk off?" We are pro-masturbation, but the type of masturbation we are advocating has little in common with the hurried, goal-oriented, tension relieving experience so aptly described by terms such as "whacking off," "jerking off," or "beating your meat."

Most males reach orgasm in one to three minutes—often as little as thirty seconds. The desire to achieve rapid ejaculation originates in early adolescence, with the fear of being caught by a parent or sibling. Adolescent boys, aware their parents disapprove of masturbation, have an understandable reluctance to linger over the experience. They want to get through quickly and dispose of the evidence before mom or dad barges in. This pattern is reinforced in the college dormitory or group living arrangement where, even though nearly every young man masturbates, none wants the others to know about it. Even when a man has privacy and the need for secrecy disappears, the habit remains. He no longer fears discovery, but has incorporated the negative views of his parents and peers. He strives to keep masturbation a secret, separate from his mature, respectable, day-to-day life.

In a literal sense, he follows the Biblical injunction "Let not thy right hand know what thy left hand doeth." By confining pleasure to the brief moments of ejaculation, he minimizes enjoyment, thus appeasing his sense of guilt. Barry's adolescent masturbatory experiences were hurried and clandestine, followed by embarrassment when he saw semen stains on his sheets.

The practice of rapid, ejaculation-oriented masturbation is another manifestation of the male machine concept. The man who stimulates his penis with the intent of "getting off" as quickly as possible is, in effect, treating himself like a sex object. But your penis is not a disembodied object. It is an integral part of you, a part of the enormously complex pattern of interacting physical and psychological components that make you a sexual human being.

Your penis is not the only part of you that is sexual. The penis has a very high concentration of nerve endings, but so do other parts of your body, including your hands, testicles, thighs, chest, anal area and face. As anyone knows who has had a massage, parts of the body whose nerve counts are relatively low, such as the back, can be extremely responsive to pleasurable sensations. Your whole body is a sex organ. Your mind is the major sex organ, with your penis a distant second. Masturbation is more than a technique to trigger brief, intense sensations localized in the penis. It can awaken the sexual potential of your entire body. Masturbation vastly increases a man's capacity for sexual awareness, which is good in and of itself as well as being valuable for partner sex.

ALLOWING YOURSELF TO EXPERIENCE MASTURBATION

The slow, sensuous, whole-body exploration and masturbation we are recommending is threatening to many men. In order to assuage guilt feelings, men tell themselves they don't masturbate for pleasurable or erotic sensations, but solely to relieve sexual tension. When you touch yourself slowly, concentrating on pleasure, you experience your body in a new way. The man's afraid uncomfortable or strange thoughts and feelings might take control. Sensuously oriented masturbation can show you parts of yourself of which you were unaware. You needn't fear this. Just as it is a truism that in order to accept love from others you must learn to respect, value, and love yourself, it is also true that in order to accept and feel comfortable with partner sex, you must learn to experience the pleasure and responsiveness of your own body.

The male concept of sexuality is unnecessarily rigid. Being aware of your body and its responses does not make you self-centered or immature. Quite the contrary, a man's failure to be a sensitive, imaginative lover can be ascribed to the fact he is not in touch with his body and pleasurable touch. By developing his capacity to experience a range of sensual and sexual touch, he will derive more pleasure than he thought possible. Equally important, heightened self-awareness will make him more conscious of his partner's sexual needs and responses.

Before we can guide and direct our partner in the kind of pleasuring that is most arousing, we need to discover and accept this for ourselves. This enhances our capacity to be receptive and responsive to the requests and responses of women. A sexually aware man who is knowledgeable about and responsible for his sexuality can sensitively share with a partner. Masturbation can serve to enhance your masculinity and self-confidence.

Arthur

Arthur provides a good example of how different mechanically oriented masturbation and pleasure-oriented masturbation can be in affecting a man's sex life. A reporter for a city newspaper, thirty-seven and divorced, Arthur had a twenty-year history of early ejaculation related to his general anxiety about sex. Ever since adolescence, Arthur masturbated frequently, rapidly and furtively. Arthur's only remembrance of his father talking to him about sex was when father said, ''If I ever catch you playing with yourself, I'll beat you silly!'' That didn't stop Arthur from masturbating, but it did increase his guilt and anxiety, as well as the speed of his response. Arthur learned and reinforced the rapid, penis oriented approach to sex and orgasm via masturbation.

In sexual experiences with women, Arthur ejaculated quickly. He had little understanding or appreciation of affectionate touching or sensual pleasuring. Arthur sought therapy to overcome the early ejaculation problem so he'd be confident in starting a new relationship. As part of therapy, he engaged in touching and self-exploration, with a temporary prohibition on orgasm. At first, he was uncomfortable, he felt silly stopping before he ejaculated. But the second time was better and the third better still. Within a month, Arthur was able to stimulate himself for a prolonged period of time and reach a high level of arousal while maintaining ejaculatory control. He learned to identify the point of ejaculatory inevitability and slow down stimulation so he could prolong arousal. He was able to stimulate himself for 7 to 10 minutes before coming to orgasm. Orgasm felt more satisfying. Pleasure-oriented masturbation increased his awareness and heightened his confidence that he would learn ejaculatory control during partner sex.

GUIDELINES FOR PLEASURE-ORIENTED MASTURBATION

Although masturbation naturally ends with orgasm, try to rid yourself of the preconception that each self-exploration experience *must* end in orgasm. Remember, we are trying to get away from the male machine concept of sexuality. Don't think of your genitals as a mechanism that must be forced to react in only one way. Focus on touching your genitals, as well as the rest of your body, in various ways and be aware of your responses. Resist the temptation to judge a particular touch as bad or good depending on whether it produces a strong erection or hastens ejaculation. Certainly, orgasm is the high point of a sexual experience. However, in order to broaden and deepen your capacity for erotic response, you can postpone the high point for the sake of exploring sensual and sexual feelings. Don't become anxious if a particular touch does not bring you closer to orgasm. We are all ejaculation addicts, and there is a tendency, when slow, whole-body stimulation is not producing a strong response, to say, "Forget this nonsense, let's get down to business with some old-fashioned pumping." Remember, just because you are not responding strongly at the moment does not mean you've lost your capacity to respond. Ejaculation is there when you want it. Relax and enjoy the sensations and feelings.

Even those who consider themselves liberal or flexible in other areas are archconservatives when it comes to masturbation. A man who orders roast beef and baked potato every time he goes to a restaurant would be considered unadventurous. But this is exactly what men do when they masturbate. The average male works out a certain technique for masturbation during early adolescence, and thereafter sticks to it until the day his penis and hand finally part company, convinced this is the only technique possible. It may surprise such diehards to learn there are virtually as many masturbation variations as there are masturbators. Masters and Johnson, who studied masturbation in a laboratory setting in their breakthrough research in 1996, found no two people used precisely the same method. And yet it rarely occurs to us to vary the technique we've become accustomed to. We seem determined not to increase the awareness and pleasure we derive from masturbation. Just as experimentation is encouraged in lovemaking, it is encouraged in masturbation.

Finally, a few words about dealing with anxiety. Some exercises may cause you to feel uncomfortable. This is understandable, the habits of a lifetime are not broken easily. If you feel anxious as a result of touching yourself in a particular place or in a particular way, don't stop stimulation. Instead, utilize a touch or movement that feels comfortable. If you halt stimulation do so with the intention to return to the exercise when the anxiety dissipates. Carry out self-exploration in slow, easy stages. Don't give in to the anxiety and return to the rigid system. The focus is to explore your body and increase awareness. Do this for yourself—you deserve to be treated gently and with respect. Any masturbation technique, as long as it's not physically harmful or compulsive, is in the normal range.

SELF-EXPLORATION/MASTURBATION EXERCISES

As adolescents we masturbate in response to sexual tension, usually without much thought about how we do it. The hand moves to the penis without conscious thought, the movements follow the well-worn tracks of a habitual pattern. This type of masturbation provides simple, uncomplicated climax. Like most habits, it moves in a tight, unvarying circle of stimulus and reward. For many men masturbation is more a response to anxiety than a pleasurable experience. We encourage you to masturbate when you are "horny" and desire a sex outlet, not to relieve boredom or anxiety. Masturbation tied to anxiety becomes a compulsive habit. There are psychologically healthier ways to deal with boredom and anxiety.

Exercise 1. To allow masturbation to be a learning experience, we must vary the pattern. Relaxation of the body and mind is essential. A leisurely bath or shower is a good way to begin. As you wash, using scented soap if you like, massage your arms, shoulders, back and legs. You probably have an inner timing device that goes off when you think the allotted time in the tub has expired. Ignore it. Give yourself permission to enjoy the experience until you feel relaxed and ready for the next phase. Be conscious of the sensations as you move from a wet environment to a dry one—the dripping of water from your body, the slight chill if it is cool, the breaking out of tiny beads of sweat if hot. Dry yourself concentrating on the feel of the towel on your skin.

Without putting on your clothes, go into the bedroom and make whatever preparations you need to feel comfortable. This includes turning down the lights, putting on music, turning on the air conditioner. Lie down on the bed in a comfortable position. Enjoy this sense of physical freedom. Remember, there is no one watching or judging how you look. You can achieve a state of relaxation by tensing the muscles in each part of your body in succession, focusing on the feelings as you release the tension. Breathe slowly, deeply, and evenly, repeating the word *relax* to yourself in rhythm with your breathing.

Roll over on your side, being aware of the way your body feels as you move. Touch yourself slowly and gently, at this point avoiding genitals. Close your eyes so you can focus on sensations. Move from feet to head, noticing how each part of your body feels. Vary the pressure of touch, the speed, and type of movement. Be aware of your response to different types of touch.

After you've explored your body through touch, try visual exploration. Look at yourself in a full-length mirror. Try to see your body objectively, the way you might look at a piece of sculpture. Instead of making judgments, such as "I'm too fat" or "My chest is too flabby," concentrate on the different parts of your body, noticing the way they fit together. You want to develop a positive, realistic body image. You could use a second mirror to view your body from the rear. Look at yourself in a way you have not done before, such as standing with your back to the mirror, bending over, and looking at your reflection through your legs.

Now focus on your genitals. Examine your penis, looking at and touching its various parts, including the glans, frenulum, and shaft. Examine your scrotum and testicles. Notice how your genitals look when you stand up, sit down, and lie down. Enhance body awareness and comfort. This may take from one to several sessions.

Exercise 2. Prepare for the second exercise with a leisurely shower or bath, followed by a few minutes of deep breathing and muscle relaxation. In this exercise, focus on specific erotic

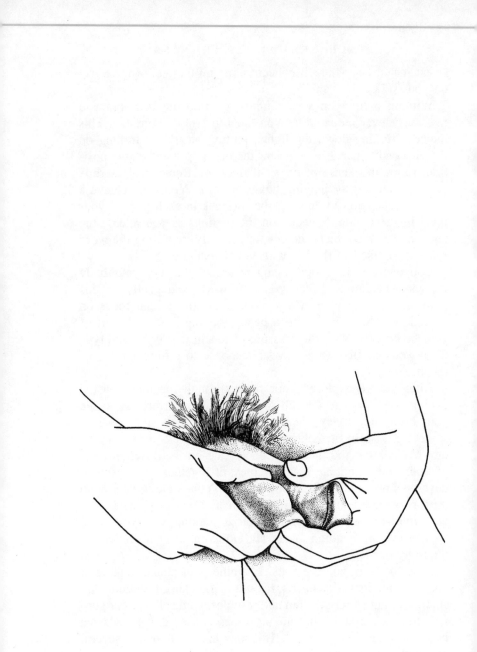

Testicular self-examination

sensations. Touch yourself in ways you find erotic and arousing. Try stimulating your nipples, which can be highly sensitive in men, just as they are in women. Notice if they become erect after stroking.

Begin stroking the insides of your thighs. Run your fingers through your pubic hair, noticing the sensations. Take your time and enjoy the range of feelings before moving your hand to your penis. Experiment with different types of penile touching and stroking to discover methods you find arousing. Try a stimulation technique you do not ordinarily use. If you use hard strokes, try gentle ones. If you are accustomed to stimulating only the glans, concentrate on movement from the shaft to the glans. Experiment with stroking and holding the testicles as well, using your other hand. Continue stimulation until you reach orgasm. The object of this exercise is to help you acquire a new awareness of and comfort with genital stimulation and erotic sensations.

Exercise 3. You can omit or include the preliminary shower, whichever you prefer. Bathing is sensual and relaxing, but there is no need to make a ritual of it. Begin with nongenital touching and caressing, noticing what feels sensuous. You may wish to experiment with erotic literature, pictures, or videos to enhance arousal. The great majority of males use fantasies during masturbation. Feel free to use written, pictorial or video material to enhance your experience. Do not fall into the trap of opting for rapid, penis oriented stimulation. Be aware, as your arousal builds, of the cycle of anticipation, desire, pleasuring, eroticism, arousal, and orgasm. Notice how your penis becomes larger and harder as arousal builds, how the glans swells and the entire genital area becomes suffused with blood. Be aware of increased muscle tension throughout your body.

Just before you begin to ejaculate, notice the intensely positive sensations at the point of ejaculatory inevitability. When you begin ejaculating one to three seconds later, concentrate on those sensations. Feel the contractions of the ejaculatory ducts, look at the semen as it spurts from your penis. After ejaculation, notice how your penis loses its erectness as you transition to the refractory phase (i.e., when you are not responsive to genital stimulation). Notice your breathing and heartrate, which sped up during arousal, return to normal levels. Do you feel sleepy or energetic after an orgasm? Examine your semen, noticing how it feels and smells. Become comfortable with it. You may even want to put a drop on your tongue to see how it tastes. The object of this exercise is to increase your acceptance and appreciation of the natural, total functioning of your body during sexual arousal.

Exercise 4. Continue experimenting with a focus on integrating sensual and sexual stimulation. Identify the kinds of stimulation that enhance your arousal. Experiment with a lubricant such as a lotion, oil, or cream. Or try masturbating by lying facedown and rubbing your penis against the sheet or pillow. You might try rolling a towel into a cylinder and inserting your penis to simulate a vagina. Try a new position or a different sequence of nongenital and genital touch. Feel free to use fantasy or erotic material as additional stimuli. Don't inhibit yourself. Feel your entire body as you enjoy erotic sensations. Focus on the most enjoyable type and amount of penile stimulation. Consistent stimulation builds the urge to ejaculate. You might experiment with a ''stop-start'' or ''slow-increase'' technique of stimulation. Allow yourself to experiment with and experience different types of penile stroking and massaging (circular, patting, heavy touch, light touch). Be aware of the point of ejaculatory inevitability, which is the beginning of the orgasm phase 1-3 seconds before you ejaculate. Let yourself go and feel the maximum of sexuality. Celebrate the full extent of your capacity for pleasure and eroticism. Orgasm is the natural culmination of high arousal and letting go.

THE POSITIVE ROLE OF MASTURBATION

Hopefully, you're clear that masturbation, far from being a ''poor excuse for the real thing,'' can be a rewarding experience in its own right. Use masturbation to enhance self-awareness and pleasure rather than as an orgasm oriented safety valve. Masturbation is an excellent way of becoming comfortable with your body and its natural and healthy responsiveness. It is amazing how, once you try sensuous, whole-body stimulation, the pleasure of the experience—no longer confined to the brief three to ten seconds of orgasm, expands into a whole new world of erotic sensations. Not only is this pleasurable in itself, but can help you share more effectively with your partner during foreplay/pleasuring intercourse, and afterplay/afterglow.

6

NEW ROLES AND CHALLENGES: CONFRONTING THE GENDER WARS

While Barry was presenting professional workshops in India, he began writing this chapter. India has a fascinating and diverse culture where marriages are arranged, males are dominant and females obedient. Traditionalists in India objected to many of the concepts presented, saying the high American premarital pregnancy rate, incidence of sexual trauma, and divorce rate proved the double-standard approach to male-female relationships is the only one that works.

We believe strongly the traditional double standard is neither workable nor preferable. It is true that the much-heralded women's movement has failed to deliver on the promise of "positive changes for women and men together." This is the time to rethink and redefine male-female relationships so they enhance psychological and sexual well-being for both sexes.

Much of the discussion of gender roles is and has been ideological, moralistic, and/or highly emotional. The "good woman-bad guy" theme dominates writing and discussion. A best selling pop psychology book emphasizes how men and women are from different planets and talk shows focus on the differences between male and female communication styles. Let us approach this multicausal, multidimensional subject from an objective, respectful, and humanistic point of view.

There has been a great deal of scientific research during the past decade examining male-female similarities and differences along a number of dimensions—physical strength, intellectual functioning, behavioral characteristics, health status, sexual response, communication of feelings, and interpersonal traits. The objective research evidence is overwhelming—there are many more similarities than differences between men and women, including the dimension of sexual response. The same phases of desire, arousal, orgasm, and emotional satisfaction are experienced by both men and women. The same psychological processes of positive anticipation and receptivity and responsivity to stimulation, the same physiological processes of arousal by vasocongestion and myotonia, the same rhythmic contractions of orgasm, and a similar resolution period occurs for men and women. Of course, there are differences, but the sexual similarities physically, psychologically, and emotionally outnumber the differences.

The two major differences involve latency of response and variability of orgasm. Women usually require a longer period of time and more direct genital stimulation for sexual arousal, although these differences decrease with age and experience. Second, male orgasmic response is more straightforward in comparison to female orgasmic response. The male will have one orgasm, which occurs during intercourse, while the woman might be nonorgasmic, singly orgasmic, or multiorgasmic. This might occur in the foreplay/pleasuring period, during intercourse, or in the afterplay/afterglow period. This does not mean female sexual response is better or worse, only more complex and variable.

The crucial similarity is men and women are sexual people with the ability to give and receive pleasure-oriented touching. Sexuality is a positive, integral part of one's personality. Men and women deserve to feel good about sexuality and for sexuality to enhance their lives and relationships.

TRADITIONAL MALE-FEMALE ROLES

Sexuality is a vital, integral component of masculinity and femininity, but not the dominant factor. In the traditional double standard, men and women are assigned dramatically different roles with little overlap. The man is socialized to play the strong, dominant role. He is the leader, the provider, the achievement-oriented person. Responsibility for the financial success of the family lies with him. He makes all the decisions outside the house. With children his role is disciplinarian. He prepares his sons for the rigors and competition of the adult, male world. For daughters, his role is protector against predatory males who only want ''one thing.'' He's responsible for making a good marriage for his daughter so she will produce grandchildren and look after the father in his old age. In terms of leisure, he has male friends to drink with, play cards with, and watch sports with. The man depends on the woman to take care of his food, clothes, and health needs. Sexually, he is the initiator, frequency is his measure of satisfaction. Sexuality is his domain and responsibility. The woman's role is to be passive, follow his lead, and have orgasms to prove he's a good lover.

In stereotypic double standard socialization, the woman takes the role of the weak, dependent spouse. Her task is to nurture and take care of her husband and children. She derives her self-esteem from their accomplishments. Her domain is the home— organizing, cooking, and cleaning. Most important, she is responsible for the family's emotional needs; she is the prime (and usually only) caretaker. Sexual pleasure is his domain, not hers. If she experiences arousal it has to be during intercourse. If she has an orgasm it has to be just like the man's—a single orgasm during intercourse. If she works outside the home, it is for extra money for the family, not to pursue her career. She is not expected to have intellectual interests. Her friends are other women and relatives. She is in charge of their social life with other couples and families. She is not to have male friends because such a relationship would undoubtedly turn into an extramarital affair (after all, why would a man want a friendship with a woman other than to have sex?).

Although readers will laugh at these rigid stereotypes and see them as outdated, they continue in a more subtle form to exert a profound effect on present day gender wars. For example, when the woman earns more money or is more sexually interested and orgasmic, this stresses the couple's relationship. Although intellectually it's supposed to be ''okay,'' ambivalent feelings (on both people's part, but especially the male's) and relationship difficulties are the norm.

Stereotyped male-female roles have a negative effect on the couple's emotional and sexual relationship. Just as important, they inhibit the personal growth of the man. Everyone, including children, lose in relationships based on these rigid, irrational roles.

It is easier to tear down an old system than develop a new model that is rational, functional, and satisfying. We do not suggest our model is perfect, or the only one, or will work for all males, all couples, or all cultures. What we propose is an equity model of male-female relationships that is congruent with scientific information about the similarities between men and women and focuses on enhancing emotional and sexual satisfaction for both sexes.

AN EQUITY MODEL OF MALE-FEMALE RELATIONSHIPS

The foundation is a respectful view of the female as a responsible, competent sexual person. The model is not one of 50-50 equality in every aspect of life (which is idealistic and doomed to failure). The 50-50 equality model does not recognize the complexities of individual attitudes, behaviors, emotions, and situations. The core of our model is equity between the man and woman. One person can have prime responsibility or skill in one area while the other has prime responsibility and skill in another area. The crucial element is the man and woman relate as respectful human beings who value each other's competence and share power in an equitable manner. You respect how you manage your life, how she manages her life, and how you relate as a couple. Caring, respectful, and equitable partners serve as excellent models for children to learn about male-female relationships. Generally, people who treat each other well outside the bedroom will treat each other well inside the bedroom.

The second dimension involves trust. Instead of men and women being at war, seeing the opposite sex as the enemy, trust your intimate partner will not do something to purposely undercut or harm you. She has your best interest in mind and is your friend and supporter. For trust to be genuine, it must be reciprocal. She needs to trust your motivations and behavior. Trust does not mean freedom from problems, disappointments, or anger. It does mean you relate in an honest manner, try to act in her best interest, and don't intentionally hurt your partner.

The third building block is intimacy and caring. Intimacy is a solid, mature basis for a relationship unlike the romantic love glorified in movies, songs and books. Romantic love is passionate and all-consuming. It offers the promise of bliss, "never having to say you're sorry." Romantic love often ends in a bitter, destructive manner. It makes great fiction, but is a self-defeating way to conduct your life. The equity model sees the choice of an intimate partner based partly in emotion, but more firmly in a realistic view of the woman (respect, trust, intimacy and communicating about a range of issues). You plan a joint life together. Your caring is deep as well as passionate. Intimacy is more than sexual, it includes sharing thoughts, feelings, beliefs, values, and plans. You deal with conflict without negating intimacy. Romantic love is only "for better." Intimate, mature love is "for better and worse." Intimate couples survive hard times, romantic love couples don't.

Sexuality is integral to an intimate relationship. Sex serves to energize the bond and make it secure. The major functions of sexuality are a shared pleasure, a means to deepen and reinforce intimacy and a tension reducer to deal with the hassles of life and the relationship. Contrary to traditional male beliefs, sex is not the most important component in a relationship. When sex goes well it's a positive integral component—15-20 percent. When sex is problematic or dysfunctional it plays an inordinately powerful role—50-75 percent, draining the relationship of good feelings and intimacy. Spouses should view each other as sexual people and sex as respectful, trusting and caring. Romantic love sex seldom lasts more than six months and no longer than two years. Intimate sex might be less frequent and intense, but is better quality and more enduring.

The ability to listen and respond empathically to your partner's thoughts and feelings is crucial. Be direct, clearly state your feelings and make requests (not demands). It is crucial to deal with problems rather than avoid them. Use problem-solving skills (stating your feelings and wants, discussing alternatives, objectively evaluating the pros and cons of each, committing to a solution, implementing the solution, and monitoring the results) and act in a constructive, focused manner. A relationship includes tolerance and humor to get past the inevitable difficult situations and hard times. Sometimes acceptance is a better strategy than change.

The most intimate and involved relationship is marriage, where these skills and attitudes play a crucial role. The equity model is relevant to work, friendships, family, and social relationships. The following are guidelines for healthy male-female relationships.

GUIDELINES FOR MALE-FEMALE RELATIONSHIPS
1. A respectful attitude toward women, viewing them as equal people.
2. An open and flexible attitude toward male-female roles.
3. An acceptance and security about yourself and your masculinity so you are not threatened or intimidated by women.
4. Awareness that intellectually, behaviorally, emotionally, and sexually there are more similarities than differences between men and women.
5. Ability to have a professional and/or personal friendship with a woman; do not sexualize male-female relationships.
6. You are comfortable and confident in your masculinity, so activities or interests that have traditionally been labeled ''feminine'' can be integrated into your life.
7. An intimate sexual relationship is more satisfying if both partners can initiate, say no, make requests and enjoy sexual pleasure.
8. An attitude that conception, contraception, and children are as much the responsibility of the man as the woman.
9. A respectful, equitable, trusting, and intimate marriage is the most satisfying.
10. Recognition that a communicative, sharing, and giving relationship promotes emotional and sexual satisfaction.

Instead of an ongoing war between the sexes, there can be mutually enhancing relationships between men and women.

Both the man and woman need to confront gender wars and stereotypes, and develop a comfortable, functional way of relating. At its base a male-female relationship is a respectful, trusting friendship where intimacy and sexuality make it special. Let us examine a couple who have chosen to implement the equity model.

Tom and Nancy

Married for eighteen years, with a fourteen-year-old daughter, these two provide a good example of the equity model in practice. Tom grew up in a working-class family characterized by a great deal of violence, including spouse and child abuse. When Tom was seven his father died in a car accident, driving while intoxicated. Mother moved the children to the medium-size city where her parents lived. Tom grew up around uncles and his grandfather, but did not have a strong male role model.

A turning point occurred in Tom's life when he was a seventeen-year-old high school junior. A freshman girl who was immature and desperately wanted attention would take boys into the woods and give "blow jobs." Tom was with three friends who were joking and bragging that this was "what life really had to offer." Tom, like most boys in his town, had been to a prostitute. In his social group being a virgin after sixteen was ridiculed. The male had to prove he wasn't a "fag." However, in viewing the scene with the freshman girl, Tom knew it was not for him. Although he wasn't assertive enough to say anything (a fact he regrets), he chose not to get involved in sexual activity where a woman is used and abused.

Tom talked to his favorite female teacher about that incident and his future plans. Good teachers earn their pay not just in the classroom, but listening to and guiding adolescents outside the classroom. She encouraged Tom to use his intellectual ability to advance himself and get a college education. A major reason students did not continue schooling or training was unwanted, unplanned pregnancies which resulted in early marriages and/or immature or abusive relationships, causing chaos and distraction in male's lives. She urged at a minimum he use condoms. For the first time, Tom was introduced to the idea that women were sexual people, not sex objects, and a dating relationship should be a respectful friendship. You trust a friend would not do anything to hurt you—shouldn't this apply to a dating and sexual relationship?

Although Tom continued to hang around with old friends, he started choosing new male and female friends who took a more serious and responsible view toward life. After graduation he attended the local community college for two years, eventually graduating from the state university. College had a positive psychological and social effect on Tom. He majored in human resource management, working summers as a clerk in a personnel department. Tom became aware of feelings engendered by being treated as a "second-class citizen" and realized even professional women were treated that way. Tom became acutely aware of the issue of sexual harassment, and its negative impact psychologically, professionally, and on company morale.

Tom resolved not to marry until he was established in his career. He enjoyed a moderately active sexual life, dating one woman at a time. Affairs lasted from six months to two years. Before beginning intercourse, he made sure she was using birth control pills, had an IUD, or used her diaphragm. If not, he always used a condom. This was before the era of HIV/AIDS where there was less awareness of the importance of safer sex strategies. Although Tom had two relationships that ended bitterly, most were good. Tom felt he had been a respectful friend and learned about himself, women and relationships.

After college, he received an assistantship to study for a master's degree in industrial relations. Nancy was in his graduate program. At first they related as professional friends because Nancy was involved in a relationship and Tom was intimidated by Nancy's academic excellence. Tom invited her to dinner after the semester ended, and they talked long into the night about personal and professional plans. Tom was aware of his sexual attraction and put in the back of his mind that he would like to date her if there was an opportunity. During the next semester, they saw each other two or three times a week as friends. Toward the end of the semester they joined a coed volleyball team. Nancy met the woman Tom was dating and he met the man Nancy was involved with. Tom wondered what attracted Nancy to this fellow, since he drank too much and treated her badly. She confided to Tom: "He treats me like shit and I don't know why I put up with it." Tom didn't either, but it took Nancy off the pedestal he'd put her on.

Dinner after semester exams was becoming a tradition. After

drinking too much wine (not a recommended behavior to initiate self-disclosure, but a common one), Tom told Nancy the story of his father's death and the teacher's advice. Nancy was a concerned listener which emboldened Tom to reveal how attracted he felt toward her. Nancy was receptive, and the evening was a romantic, sensuous one—but did not culminate in intercourse. The next day Tom called and invited her for a walk in the park. Tom told her his feelings of the previous night were genuine, that it was not the wine talking. If they were to become a romantic couple, Tom wanted Nancy to first make a clean break from her current boyfriend. He didn't want a messy scene where he would try to take her away and she would vacillate between the two men. Nancy was angry because she hoped a new relationship would give her the impetus to get out of the self-defeating one. However, she realized Tom was right, it was her responsibility to break off the affair, she should not use Tom as an excuse. It took Nancy a full six weeks to terminate the relationship. During that time Tom continued to be supportive, not coercing or issuing ultimatums.

Once they began as a romantic and sexual couple, it was passionate and fun. They did the special things lovers do—stay up for hours talking, spend the next day in bed making love, eat popcorn for breakfast, make love at midnight on the beach, and dream of the perfect marriage and life. Romantic love is an experience not to be missed, but at best it only lasts a year or two. Romantic love is not a basis for marriage.

After graduation Tom and Nancy did two hard, but necessary, tasks. They visited each other's families and talked frankly about the elements in their backgrounds they admired and wanted to emulate and elements that were "traps" (i.e., problems they would have to be careful to monitor and avoid). For Tom, the trap was playing the dominant role and looking at the woman as "weak, pure, and having to be taken care of." Nancy came from an alcoholic family where her stepbrother had sexually abused her between ages eleven and thirteen. She had a hard time trusting men. Although she was professionally self-confident, her trap was personal and sexual self-esteem was dependent on the approval of the man.

A healthy relationship brings out the best in each person. Nancy wanted Tom to acknowledge he was competent, someone who could work with others in a respectful, cooperative manner rather than dominate them. Tom wanted Nancy to see herself as a survivor, not a victim. She could trust herself and trust him. She needed to build personal and sexual self-esteem on a broad, solid foundation.

The second hard task was to decide about career issues and where to live. The old system in which the man's career always came first did not promote male-female equity, but it was easier. It is difficult to coordinate two careers, especially when both people are in the same field. Tom and Nancy agreed to look at a range of alternatives and make decisions that took into account both career and personal needs. They were not so naive to believe all decisions would be equal or easy. They chose to look for jobs in the three large cities they wanted to live. Each had a veto power—although Tom would have liked New York, Nancy found it too expensive and hectic. Nancy liked the idea of Dallas or Houston, but Tom wanted to avoid Texas for work-related reasons. They settled on Washington, D.C.

This concept of each having a veto power over important life decisions has served them well. For instance, six years into their marriage, Tom was interested in having a second child, but Nancy vetoed the idea since she felt with their careers, activities, and marital bond a second child would decrease the quality of their lives and family. A hard decision, but raising a child entails a strong, mutual commitment from both people. Tom realized he could not force Nancy to have a second child.

Tom and Nancy had a strong commitment to making the marriage satisfying and secure. They would not stay in a destructive marriage for tradition, dependency, or the sake of their child. This agreement reinforced the commitment to keep their marital bond respectful, trusting, and intimate. They would not take the marriage for granted and allow it to stagnate. Sexuality plays an integral role in energizing their marriage and maintaining emotional connection.

A marriage (and marital sex) needs consistent attention and commitment to growth. As Nancy and Tom changed as individuals, their marriage needed to be cohesive and flexible to adjust to personal changes. For a marriage to thrive both people have to be good listeners, be clear and direct in stating opinions and making requests, look at a range of alternatives when facing a problem, and make decisions in a respectful manner so they reach an agreement both can live with. The latter has been crucial in terms of balancing career issues and raising their child. Tom would have preferred Nancy to have been a more traditional, less ambitious professional. However, he had to admit her influence and questioning made him a more aware and involved professional, unlike colleagues who "burned-out" in their jobs by age forty. The security of a second income allowed Tom to take professional risks (i.e., start his own consulting firm, which he might not have done if he were the primary or sole provider). On the other hand, he regretted not having the flexibility to change locations for a better job opportunity. Life is a series of problem-solving challenges where you make the best decision based on realistic alternatives, not an ideal world where you have total control and can have it all.

Tom was more involved in the nitty-gritty tasks of parenting than he ever imagined he would be. From changing diapers, to going to school open houses, to taking his daughter shopping, to talking to her about friendships, Tom was a nurturing father. He found parts of parenting aggravating, such as driving car pools and waiting around, but other parts tremendously gratifying, such as helping her prepare for her first dance (Nancy was out of town on business). Tom felt sorry for male friends who were only marginally involved in parenting.

Tom and Nancy had a vital sexual relationship, based on a broad-based, flexible approach to touching and eroticism. Although Tom was more likely to initiate intercourse, Nancy was just as likely to initiate pleasuring and playing together. Nancy was orgasmic during intercourse using multiple stimulation, but found it easier and more satisfying being orgasmic during nonintercourse sex, especially manual stimulation. Nancy and Tom would have a pleasuring date at least once every three months to experiment and play with nongoal-oriented touching. Nancy and Tom were affectionate on a daily basis, sensual every other day, and sexual 1-3 times a week. Touching and sexuality energized their marital bond and enhanced feelings of being a special couple.

As Tom and Nancy look toward the future, they're aware life will present them with challenges and change. They spend time talking, planning, and developing goals for the second part of their lives. They look forward to launching their daughter into college and have no fear of an "empty nest" syndrome. They plan to pursue individual interests—Tom to write a book advocating progressive policies concerning maternity/paternity leave and flexible work hours and Nancy to run for the city council. Tom hopes to pursue his interest in hiking (which Nancy shares) and his hobby of golf, while Nancy pursues her interest in gardening. They plan to travel and do social justice projects with their church group.

INDIVIDUALIZING AN EQUITABLE RELATIONSHIP

Human beings, sexuality and relationships are too complex and individualistic for hard rules which apply to all men and situations. Be aware of, individualize and implement these guidelines for an equitable relationship. Male-female relationships should be based on respecting the woman and relating in a trustful, nondominating manner. The double standard needs to be challenged—personally, relationally, sexually and culturally. In developing equitable relationships (especially a sexually intimate relationship), the man has as much to learn from the woman as she has to learn from him. In a healthy relationship, both the man and woman are comfortable talking about feelings, comfortable with affectionate and sensual touch, both can sexually initiate, say no or offer an alternative; and value eroticism, intercourse, orgasm, and afterplay/afterglow. In an equitable relationship, sexuality is integrated into their lives and marital bond.

7

TOUCHING, PLEASURING, INTERCOURSE, AND AFTERPLAY

How important is a hug? A kiss? A caress? If you are like most men, you rate these low on the scale of activities which are essential to your happiness.

You didn't always think that way. When you were a baby your need for affection was as vital as the food you ate or the air you breathed. If you had suddenly been deprived of physical contact, the effect would have been almost as devastating as the absence of food or oxygen. Babies do not develop normally ("failure to thrive" syndrome) if they do not regularly receive physical warmth and affection. To an infant, caring touch is essential nourishment.

Affection, besides being a source of pleasure, means the child is loved. We never lose our need for physical warmth and caring, nor should we. Whether we are eight or eighty, it is nice to be touched.

TOUCH DEPRIVATION IN MALES

Unfortunately, as boys grow older, we touch and are touched less and less. From a very early age, boys receive far less physical affection than girls. This is part of traditional socialization to make males strong, tough, self-reliant, even stoic, to prepare us for the rigors of adult competition. Frankly, there is no evidence to support this male training program. In fact, it results in decreased psychological and sexual well-being for males.

Men regard sexuality as competitive and goal-oriented, the

goal being intercourse. The man who "scores" is regarded with admiration by male friends, and the one who scores with many women is accorded special respect and envy. In sex, the goal is orgasm; this brief, intense sensation is considered the only really worthwhile part of sex. The average man begins as an early ejaculator, but even when he learns to prolong lovemaking (the average length of intercourse is 2 to 7 minutes), he does so for the benefit of the woman. As for the physical expressions of affection that precede intercourse, the very name—foreplay—conveys these are mere preliminaries to the "real thing."

Selling short pleasurable experiences is self-defeating. We dismiss kisses, hugs, and spontaneous caresses as having little value if not followed by intercourse and orgasm. Women place a higher value on pleasuring which reflects the greater freedom they are permitted in expression of touching and affection. This disparity between the value men and women place on affection and pleasuring is a frequent source of contention and misunderstanding.

TOUCHING

Women are dissatisfied with the amount of intimate contact and affection they receive from their partners. Men are confused by this criticism because it is difficult to think of affection and/or sensuality as worthwhile in itself. Men regard the expression of love as a specialized activity, circumscribed spatially by the four walls of the bedroom and temporally by the time between lights-out and sleep. For men, touching is goal-oriented.

We have imposed on ourselves a state of sensual impoverishment. By opening ourselves to nondemand pleasuring, we can regain the rich and rewarding world of touch. Affectionate touch conveys not only a sense of contact, security, and comfort but emotions such as caring, gratitude, and desire. Affection involves clothes on touching such as holding hands, kissing, and hugging. Sensuality involves touching when you're semi-clothed or nude, including caressing, whole body massage, nongenital pleasuring, bathing or showering together, cuddling in bed for 10 minutes before going to sleep or on awakening. Sensuality is a way to feel connected and share pleasure.

Men narrowly define sexual pleasure as the sensations expe-

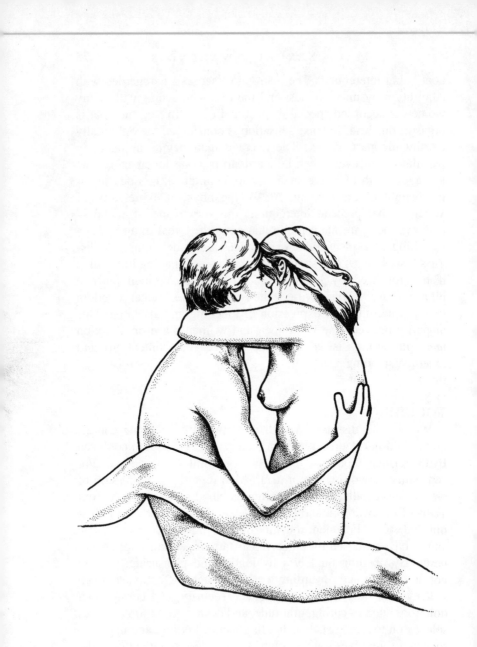

Giving and receiving pleasurable touching is the core of sexual responsiveness.

rienced through the genitals during intercourse. This definition negates affectionate touching, sensual pleasuring, and erotic stimulation. What about the pleasure of seeing our partner's body, either nude or in various stages of undress? The pleasure of whispered words of love, or the excitement of hearing your partner's moans and breathing? The smells of your partner's body mingling with yours? The sense of movement as we engage in erotic stimulation? The tastes experienced during oral sex? What of the myriad ways a couple can share pleasure?

Nor is pleasure limited to the bedroom. For example, there is the exquisite thrill of touching knees or hands under a table. There is the erotic reaction to sniffing a particular perfume. What about the pelvic sensations we experience in response to a certain phrase spoken in a certain tone of voice? We can be sensual and sexual people throughout the day, pleasure may occur anytime, anywhere. We can be receptive through all our senses. It's folly to limit sex to a strictly delineated time and place (the bedroom at night) and to a specific range of physical sensations (the penis, intercourse, and the three to ten seconds of orgasm). Our mind is the ultimate sex organ, determining what feelings, sensations, and touches we are receptive and responsive to.

PLEASURING AND INTERCOURSE

Unfortunately, our mind acts as a censor, closing pleasurable circuits, forbidding nongoal-oriented feelings and sensations. Touching, caressing, and kissing are most exciting at the beginning of a relationship. He is learning how she expresses herself, and anticipates further exploration and touching. Discovering new things about your partner is exciting. For couples who have not yet had intercourse, fantasies about sex are rich and varied.

When a couple has intercourse regularly, touching and affection lose their significance. Intercourse becomes the primary or sole means of physical connection. Kissing and caressing, once so exciting and important, are now mere "foreplay," a brief, hurried prelude to coitus. What began as nondemand, pleasure-oriented touching gives way to goal-oriented foreplay.

Intercourse is central to sexual expression, but there is something very wrong with the idea that affectionate, sensual, and erotic touch is worthwhile only when followed by intercourse.

If intercourse is to remain satisfying, there must be experimentation, spontaneity, and variety. Trying new intercourse positions is one way of introducing creativity into the sexual relationship, but there are countless ways of expressing pleasure through affectionate, sensual, and erotic experiences. If we are to introduce new energy and enjoyment, what better way than to reopen our closed circuits, expand our consciousness, open up a new world of sensual and sexual experiences? Sometimes this will lead to intercourse, and other times it may be a way of communicating pleasure, playfulness, or sensuality.

An analogy couples find helpful is to a 5-speed car. Gear 1 is clothes on affectionate touching. Gear 2 is nongenital pleasuring, a sensual experience which can be semi-clothed or nude. Gear 3 is playful touch, usually nude, which involves genital as well as nongenital pleasuring. Gear 4 is erotic stimulation (manual, oral, or rubbing stimulation) to high levels of arousal and orgasm (nonintercourse sex). Gear 5 involves intercourse and orgasm. Although most rides will involve all 5 gears, it isn't necessary. Sometimes you just want a leisurely drive in the country. Each touching gear has value in itself. Every touching experience needn't go to Gear 5 to justify starting the car. Enjoy each affectionate, pleasuring, and erotic experience for itself.

One reason we've lost our capacity to experience pleasure is we've become too serious and goal-oriented. As adolescents, we responded intensely because each experience was new. We allowed ourselves to be curious and involved. But as we matured, we assumed our knowledge was complete. We knew all there was to know sexually. If we could recapture openness of mind and senses, we would find the world is full of novel and surprising experiences. Ways of expressing affection are almost limitless, part of the fun is discovering new activities that are sensual and pleasurable.

SENSUALITY GUIDELINES

These guidelines encourage you to explore the world of touching and sensuality. You can increase awareness of ordinary acts of touching such as hand contact. Pick up your partner's hand and spend some time examining it as though you are seeing it for the first time. Turn her hand over and trace the lines of the

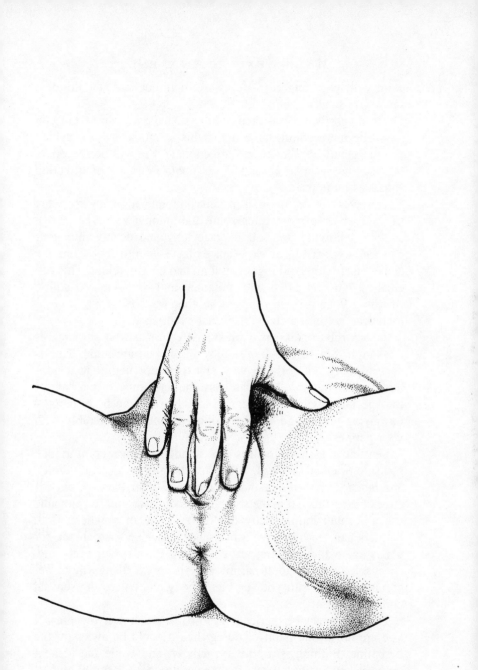

He can learn to be comfortable giving erotic stimulation.

palm with your fingertip. Be aware of the delicate tactile messages you send to your partner.

We suggest setting aside time for sensual exploration, but you might be more comfortable doing this spontaneously. Provided you are genuinely tender and affectionate, she will be receptive. In fact, the surprise caused by a spontaneous act of affection enhances its impact.

The eyes are organs of sensual communication. In everyday life, we observe strict rules about the amount and type of eye contact. Allowing yourself to gaze long and deeply into your partner's eyes can be an experience of special intimacy. Combine eye contact with touching, caressing, and hand-holding. This can create a moment filled with poignant and romantic sensuality. Brushing your partner's hair is another way of turning a commonplace act into a shared, sensual experience.

A back rub or massage expresses affection as well as increases relaxation. Massage is more enjoyable if you are nude. This is an especially comfortable way to experience nudity in a non-intercourse situation. You can learn the fine points of massage— the special movements designed to relax specific body parts— by buying a massage book or taking a course—preferably with your partner.

Sensual massage focuses on nondemanding, comfortable, pleasure oriented feelings. Allow touching to be slow, rhythmic, and tender, with no demand for response other than the experience of pleasure. To make sensual massage even more enjoyable use a scented lotion (baby oil, body lotion, or powder). Both partners can learn to give a massage. Either person can ask for a massage without feeling self-conscious. Besides being relaxing, enjoyable, and invigorating, massage is an excellent way of becoming at ease with your partner's body and enhancing sensual communication.

Another sensual experience is to bathe or shower together. If you are not in the habit of doing this, it could be awkward the first time. Bathing is a solitary activity, and while the idea of doing it with a partner may be appealing, there is initial embarrassment. The next time she takes a bath, say, "Do you mind if I join you?" If she has a splitting headache and wants to spend a quiet hour in a warm tub, accept a no. If the initial response is based on self-consciousness, say, "Come on, it'll be fun," or

"We don't have to do anything except enjoy a bath together." Showering or bathing is a sensual, relaxing experience and a nice way to explore touching. Take turns slowly soaping each other. The addition of warm water and rich, soapy lather enhances sensual feelings. Extend the pleasure by slowly drying each other. Showering or bathing is excellent preparation for mutual pleasuring, oral sex, and/or intercourse. It is a wonderful way of becoming relaxed and open to physical sensations. It has the advantage of making the body clean and sweet-smelling so it is a particular pleasure to touch and be touched.

Steve

Steve thought of himself as a "new man," liberated from the restraints of the traditional male role. He'd been married five years to Susan, had a two-year-old daughter, and was an involved parent. Because of time demands, sex occurred late at night after their daughter was asleep. Although both Steve and Susan were playful and affectionate with their child, they had fallen into a nonaffectionate couple pattern.

One night they had a fire in the fireplace, and their child curled up and fell asleep. As Steve and Susan were basking in the glow of the fire, Steve became aware how much he missed these experiences. As a premarital couple, and early in the marriage, they had been affectionate and playful. Both looked back fondly on their courtship, when they would cuddle on the couch for an hour; shower together and sometimes be sexual in the shower; engage in long, sensual touching that culminated in intercourse; and regularly exchange hugs. Steve shared with Susan how disappointed he was they had allowed this aspect of their lives to wither.

Susan challenged Steve's assumption it had to be that way. They put their daughter to bed and returned to the fire. Steve found the next hour and a half the most enjoyable of the past year. They talked, hugged, caressed, recalled memories, and thoroughly enjoyed a very sensuous time. It culminated in intercourse since both felt turned-on and aroused. Even if they had stayed with sensual play, it would have been a very special experience.

The next day Steve and Susan went for a walk and vowed

they would revitalize affection and sensuality. Affection and sensuality was a vital part of their life that had slipped away. They realized the prior night was special and could not be easily duplicated. They looked forward to touching both inside and outside the bedroom as a way of reaffirming their caring and love. In addition, they began doing whole-family hugs. Steve valued affectionate and sensual time as a way of connecting with Susan as well as building sexual anticipation.

OTHER FUNCTIONS OF TOUCH

Affectionate and sensual expression conveys caring and tenderness. Yet, touching has many potential functions. Relationships have a degree of frustration and tension built into them. It is better to express such feelings rather than let them fester. There are many ways to do this, including a pillow fight, wrestling, or a tickling match. These can be stimulating as well as provide an emotional release. It's healthy as long as you do not use sex as a way to express anger. Tension reduction to deal with the frustrations of life and marriage is a valid function for touching and sexuality.

Feel free to express yourself in ways that seem childish or foolish. You can play artificial roles, indulging in fantasy and pantomime. Some common roles include the princess with the slave, the sultan with the harem girl, and the adventurer with the shy virgin. You recognize these are fantasies, so feel free to play and express yourself.

Imagination, sensitivity, and a willingness to try new activities are qualities which expand our pleasure quotient. The pleasure to be derived from spontaneous, novel, affectionate, and sensual experiences is a substantial reward in its own right. In addition, this will have a positive effect on the quality of your sex life.

THE FUNCTIONS OF SEX

Unlike the sex habits of animals, the sexual behavior of human beings is not controlled by instinctual or biological factors. Human sexuality is a function of psychological, relational, and cultural factors. It is this capacity for learning and choice that facilitates variety in human sexual expression. Sex for procreation is a rare occurrence among humans. We have sex for pleasure, to express love, as a tension reducer, as a form of communication, for warmth, and to reinforce and deepen intimacy. Sex between humans is far more complex and emotionally significant.

While it seems obvious human sex is much superior to animal sex, many men haven't heard the news yet. Some of us have barely gotten past the animal stage of lovemaking. Men are addicted to sexual expression that is goal oriented, penis oriented, intercourse oriented, and orgasm oriented. Many of us, like animals, think of sex as something we do to a female. This attitude is reflected in slang expressions, such as "I laid her" or "I made her." Other men have been persuaded by sex articles and talk shows that a woman's sexual responses are slower and she needs stimulation to make her "ready" for intercourse. It is his job to make sure he "gives her an orgasm"—like a work order to be filled.

Men think of nonintercourse stimulation as being exclusively for the woman, having little meaning or pleasure for them. But, neither *to* nor *for* accurately describes what sexuality can be. A better word and attitude is *with*. Both the male body and the female body are enormously complex structures, gloriously endowed with the capacity to experience pleasure. The most satisfying sex is intimate and interactive, two people giving and receiving pleasure-oriented touch. This is the core of human sexuality, not only for women but equally for men.

MALE AND FEMALE SIMILARITIES AND DIFFERENCES

Male and female sexual response involves more similarities than differences. Men and women need to think of each other as sexual people equally capable of experiencing desire, arousal, orgasm, and emotional satisfaction. But there is a major difference: female sexual response is more variable and complex— not better or worse. The woman may be nonorgasmic, singly orgasmic, or multiorgasmic, which can occur during any phase (pleasuring, intercourse, or afterplay) of the sexual experience. The male typically has a single orgasm which occurs during intercourse.

The title of this chapter—"Touching, Pleasuring, Intercourse, and Afterplay"—emphasizes the fact that there is more to sex than "getting it in and getting it off." Intercourse—that part of sex between intromission and ejaculation—is the high point, but it is not the be-all and end-all of sexuality. It is, rather, one of the many activities in which partners give and receive pleasure. Intercourse is more satisfying if we allow ourselves to freely explore and enjoy the range of sensual and sexual expression surrounding it. Intercourse is best conceptualized as a pleasuring technique, special and integral, but not separate from the pleasuring process. A typical lovemaking session is between 20 and 45 minutes, of which intercourse takes 2-7 minutes.

We describe pleasuring, intercourse, and afterplay as separate aspects of sexual expression. Each phase is characterized by its own distinct feelings as well as some that are common to all three. Each can be enjoyable in its own right, for its own sake, as well as part of the sexual process. The three phases may be enjoyed in different combinations, depending on the feelings of the couple and limitations imposed by the situation. Pleasuring may lead to intercourse or be engaged in for its own sake. On occasion, intercourse may begin at once, without any prelude. Afterplay may follow intercourse or be dispensed with—according to the wishes and needs of the couple. The three phases will be considered separately but with the awareness that, like courses of a fine meal, they are best combined to form a satisfying sexual experience.

PLEASURING

The term traditionally used to describe the sensual and erotic activities that precede intercourse is *foreplay*. We prefer *pleasuring,* and there is a good reason for this shift in terminology. *Foreplay* suggests something that derives its significance from what follows. Just as it is difficult to conceive of a foreword without the book it is meant to introduce, it is difficult to think of foreplay as anything but a prelude to intercourse. Foreplay, as presented in most sex manuals, is a procedure whose purpose is to arouse the woman, to bring her to the same pitch of excitement as the man. The problem is not with the activity, but with the attitude and spirit in which it is undertaken. The man engages in foreplay to fulfill an obligation. The woman experiences self-consciousness because he is doing it for her and she better get aroused as fast as possible. This performance pressure and goal orientation cheats both of pleasure.

Pleasuring, on the other hand, is a mutual activity. It refers to the feelings and behaviors a couple engage in to facilitate sensual and sexual enjoyment. Pleasuring is not goal-oriented; it is a nondemand activity engaged in for its own sake. Pleasuring can lead to feeling turned on and culminate in intercourse. But this need not be a demand or pressure. Pleasuring experiences that are not followed by intercourse can be particularly tantalizing and erotic. Barry and Emily engage in a pleasuring session every 4-6 weeks in which we agree beforehand not to proceed to intercourse, no matter how aroused we feel. This provides an excellent way to reexplore our sensual and erotic responses and reinforce variety and novelty in our sexual relationship.

Pleasuring is particularly important for men since most of us pay little attention to the nuances of our feelings. We are well acquainted with the pleasure of intercourse and orgasm, but are unaware of what else makes us feel good. We rate the value of our responses in terms of intensity. Since orgasm is the most intense sensation, we are orgasm oriented. Increasing awareness of sensual and sexual feelings will increase our enjoyment. To do this, we need to change our approach. There is more to a man's body than his penis, more to sex than intercourse, and more to satisfaction than the three to ten seconds of orgasm. Developing sensitivity to a broad range of sensual and erotic stimuli is one of the best favors you can do for yourself. This heightened awareness is extremely beneficial for your intimate relationship.

The most difficult concept for men to accept is the nongoal orientation of pleasuring. Men (and women) place an implicit demand on themselves that every erotic encounter must culminate in intercourse and orgasm. Fulfilling this requirement becomes a matter of pride, a test of masculinity. When a sexual encounter does not end in intercourse and orgasm, he feels something is wrong. Or he considers nondemand, nongoal-oriented touching as immature, reminiscent of adolescent sessions of necking and petting. But if you are honest, you remember how much you enjoyed those experiences. There is no reason why you shouldn't enjoy them again, even more so, since maturity and the comfort of a relationship allows you greater intimacy and experimentation. Men feel each encounter culminating with intercourse and orgasm is a right they have earned by becoming adults. What they forget is true maturity means freedom, the right to choose, the ability to be self-directing. The mature person can choose not to press for intercourse, instead enjoy sensual pleasure or experience orgasm through manual, rubbing, or oral stimulation.

Pleasuring Exercises. The variety of pleasuring techniques are endless. These guidelines are drawn from exercises used by couples in sex therapy. Give yourselves at least half an hour free of interruptions. Take the phone off the hook or put the answering machine on. Make whatever preparations you like to set the mood. Turn the lights in your bedroom down (but not off—you want to see what you're doing) or light a candle. Put your favorite CD on the stereo or burn incense. We have a scented candle in our bedroom that creates just the right sensual atmosphere, but the choice of such paraphernalia depends on individual tastes.

An excellent technique to structure the pleasuring experience is to designate one partner as the giver and the other as the recipient. These roles are arbitrary and might be determined by flipping a coin. The role of the recipient is to accept pleasure. This is harder than it sounds. Males find the recipient role more difficult because they are not used to being passive sexually. Close your eyes during the experience. This makes it easier to focus on sensations and reduce whatever self-consciousness you or your partner may feel. The giver's role is to give pleasure, to explore and learn about the partner's body. The first time, engage in nongenital touching. Explore sensual as opposed to sexual stimulation. The recipient is receptive to a wide variety of sensual experiences to discover what is most comfortable and pleasurable. The giver is free to use hard and light touching, kissing, licking, biting, barely touching with the fingertips, or any other technique he finds enjoyable.

Switch during the pleasuring session so each partner experiences both roles. As the couple becomes comfortable with pleasuring concepts and techniques, the process becomes mutual and interactive, more spontaneous and less structured.

Begin with the recipient lying facedown. The giver can stroke and caress the partner from head to toe, experimenting with different kinds of touching, kissing, massaging, all the while being aware of the look and feel of her body. The recipient turns over and the giver continues touching and exploring the front of the body. Looking at your partner's body is an important part of pleasuring. Begin pleasuring sessions with nongenital touching. In subsequent pleasuring sessions, stimulate the breasts and genitals. Many men are highly sensitive in the breast and nipple area; you may not have been aware of this because you mistakenly believed only the woman's breast is an "erogenous zone." An interesting variation is for both partners to keep their eyes closed. This has the effect of heightening other senses, making you aware of feelings you might otherwise miss.

Looking and touching increases awareness, especially of your partner's genitals. Many men are not aware of the clitoris or don't realize direct clitoral stimulation can be irritating and even painful. Most women prefer stimulation around the clitoral shaft and inner lips (labia minora). Let your partner guide you, she is the expert on her body and sexual responsivity.

In subsequent pleasuring sessions, the recipient can participate actively by putting his hands over hers and guiding to areas that are particularly sensitive. Show her the kind of touch which is most arousing. Nonverbal guidance is particularly effective. Sometimes the difference between a pleasant and unpleasant sensation may be a fraction of an inch to the right or left or a bit more or less pressure. Keep your eyes open and use visual contact to communicate receptivity and responsiveness. If something the partner does produces discomfort, the recipient should not call a halt, but suggest an alternative pleasuring activity. If the giver notices stress or uneasiness, he shouldn't stop, but return to an activity that is comfortable. Negative feedback can be incorporated without interrupting the sensual flow.

There are many excellent positions for pleasuring—in fact, more than for intercourse. For example, the giver sits upright with his back against the wall or headboard with legs spread apart. The recipient sits with her back leaning against his chest. This allows full access to her body, and makes it easy for her to guide his hands to those areas which are particularly sensitive. She can demonstrate the kind of touch which is most arousing.

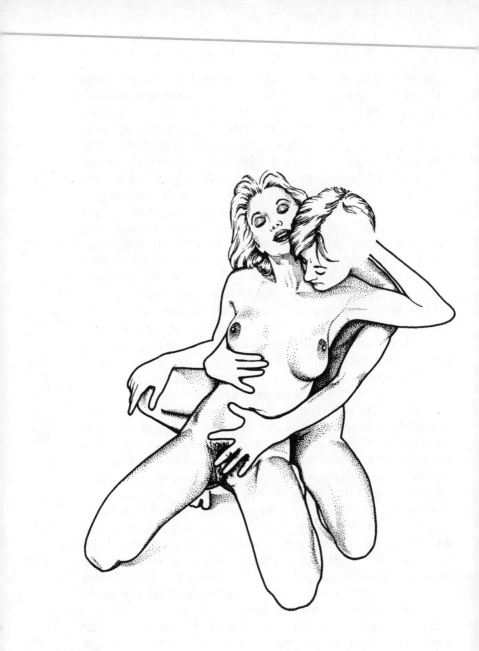

An illustration of creative positions for sexual exploration and mutual erotic pleasure.

Pleasuring can be enhanced through the use of emollients such as baby oil, hand lotion, or powder. Choose one with a smell and texture you find sensuous. Feel free to use any technique your imagination suggests so long as it is stimulating and fun. Experiment with external turn-ons—anything from a vibrator to a feather. Remember, an erection is not a sign pleasuring should end and intercourse begin. When an erection occurs, enjoy it, but you do not have to do anything about it. On the other hand, don't feel alarmed if you do not get an erection. Pleasuring is an exercise in whole-body stimulation and response. Your penis is just part of the big sex organ known as the human body.

INTERCOURSE

There is not a sharp dividing line between pleasuring and intercourse. Pleasuring does not stop when intercourse starts. Multiple stimulation such as kissing, caressing, breast stimulation, clitoral stimulation, anal stimulation, and testicle stimulation can continue during intercourse. Intercourse is a special form of pleasuring. It is an activity in which a couple gives each other pleasure through the intromission and movement of the penis in the vagina while continuing erotic stimulation.

Thinking about intercourse in this way can be an eye-opening experience. The average intercourse lasts between two to seven minutes, and orgasm takes three to ten seconds of that time. Intercourse need not be a mad rush to orgasm. An occasional "quickie" is highly exciting and satisfying. However, when "quickies" constitute the entirety of a couple's sexual repertoire, the result is monotony, frustration, and eventually resentment on the woman's part. When the man learns to take his time, to savor the sexual experience, he will find there are a thousand nuances of pleasure to be enjoyed along the way. Orgasm is still waiting faithfully at the end of the line—and usually better after the slow, tantalizing buildup.

Men think of sexual arousal as a steady drive to intercourse and orgasm. Actually, there are four phases in the sexual arousal cycle: excitement, plateau, orgasm, and resolution. In the excitement phase, the penis becomes erect and the testes are elevated. As stimulation continues, the male enters the plateau phase, where excitement increases, his erection becomes firmer, breathing becomes heavier, skin breaks out in a "sex flush." Intercourse begins either at the end of the excitement phase or during the plateau phase. Males are used to going to intercourse on their first erection. Although there is nothing wrong with this, be aware it's not the only scenario. Intensity of stimulation (both physical and psychological) is what determines arousal. If he is consistently stimulated, without pause, he progresses through the excitement and plateau phases and reaches ejaculation quickly. If, however, you vary the amount and intensity of stimulation, you can experiment with variations in the pattern and time of arousal.

PROLONGING INTERCOURSE

How can you introduce changes in the arousal and intercourse process? What can you do to prolong intercourse? There are many folk remedies for early ejaculation, such as biting hard on the corner of the pillow or fixing your mind on something unpleasant or anti-erotic. These methods are effective in reducing the intensity of stimulation, but at what cost? The feeling of a pillow between your teeth or the thought of income tax payments add nothing to the erotic experience. Using these methods causes you to resent the partner, feeling you are depriving yourself of pleasure for her sake. It serves as a distraction, which could cause arousal to decrease and mark the beginning of erection problems.

There is a much better way of achieving ejaculatory control. The first step is to discard the demand for quick arousal and orgasm. Although it sounds counterintuitive, focus on the stimulation you are experiencing. The more fully you focus on the sensations of intercourse and are comfortable with the nuances of pleasure, the less intense will be the demand for orgasm, the longer the experience will last, and the more pleasurable.

The difference in approach is between a sprinter straining to reach the finish line and a person strolling at a leisurely pace through a lovely, enthralling countryside, using all his senses to take in as much of the experience as possible. Enjoy the sexual journey as well as the arrival.

The man learns to recognize the point of ejaculatory inevitability, at which he loses voluntary control and will ejaculate. Once you've identified the point of ejaculatory inevitability, reduce the amount of stimulation before the point is reached, allowing arousal and intercourse to be prolonged. The focus is on pleasure rather than performance, making intercourse more enjoyable for you and your partner (more detail is provided in Chapter 14—"Learning Ejaculatory Control").

VARIETY IN POSITIONS

Variety is important. Of the many possible intercourse positions, couples use male on top exclusively or almost exclusively. There is nothing wrong with this position: it is comfortable, intromission is easy, the penis seldom slips out, and, since you're facing each other, it allows you to kiss and caress freely. Other intercourse positions, however, offer unique advantages.

The point of trying a variety of positions is not to prove yourself a sexual contortionist. It is to introduce a sense of novelty and discovery, which is as important in sex as other aspects of life. Discovering and sharing a new restaurant, hobby, friend, book, movie, or new way of making love can enrich and deepen your experience. Just as rigidity and monotony have a deadly effect on other activities, it has a dampening influence on the couple's sex life, making sex a mechanical habit.

This book is not meant to be a sex manual, so we will not describe other positions, the most common of which are female on top, side by side, and rear entry. For optimal sexual pleasure a couple are free to experiment and choose positions they find comfortable and stimulating. Two or three positions become your favorites. Others require a particular mood so you utilize them only on occasion. Others you use rarely, when you are feeling especially adventurous. But you will never build this repertoire unless you experiment and find which positions suit you and which do not.

Introduce variety in the type of coital thrusting. Men rely primarily on rapid in-and-out thrusting where they control the rhythm. Experiment with circular, up and down, or slow, tantalizing movement. The woman can set the tempo, rather than the male always controlling thrusting. Try a minimal, slow movement (the "quiet vagina" exercise) to enjoy feelings of vaginal

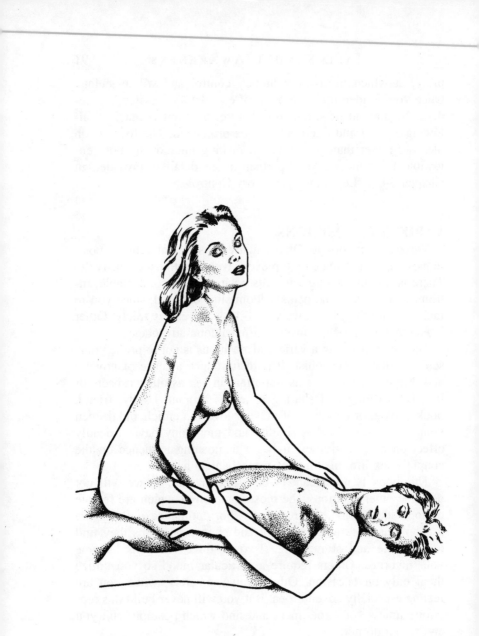

The woman astride the man while both continue caressing each other. Varying positions and erotic stimulation during intercourse enhances satisfaction.

containment. Try a rhythm that increases in tempo and then holds steady.

Another element where variety is important is who is initiator. Usually it's the man, a holdover from dating patterns. There is no rational reason why this should be the norm. A reversal of traditional roles can be a turn-on for both partners. The most satisfying relationship is one in which both partners feel free to initiate and both are free to say no or offer an alternative. The key is developing an open attitude toward sexual scenarios and techniques.

Just as there are times when you experience such urgent sexual desire that you feel like pouncing on your partner, there are times she feels the same way about you. Instead of being intimidated, accept and enjoy it. Men are distracted by worrying whether they'll get an erection when the partner initiates. Female initiation is not a demand for immediate performance, it's an invitation for sexual pleasuring. As long as you are receptive and responsive, erection and intercourse will be there. If the man is not aroused or interested in intercourse at that time, he can say no and suggest another pleasuring activity. Remember, sexuality is about pleasure, not performance.

AFTERPLAY

Afterplay (also called afterglow) is the most neglected phase of the sexual experience. The phase following orgasm has been characterized as a negative state, an anticlimactic time. This is utter nonsense. There is absolutely no physiological reason for this phase of sex to be awkward or unhappy. It can be a very pleasurable time. Both partners bask in feelings of relaxation and satisfaction, savoring the nuances of their bodily sensations. Afterplay is the experiential component of the fourth stage of sexual response, the resolution phase. Although the penis returns to the flaccid state rather quickly, the entire resolution phase entails a considerable amount of time. In a young man, vasocongestion may take three to four hours to disappear completely; in an older man, it's about a half hour.

Men assume sex is over with orgasm and the only possible activities are to get up and go about their business or fall asleep. The first pattern is the result of early experiences with clandestine lovemaking, when it was important to quickly erase all evidence of sex for fear of discovery. The second pattern is a conditioned response based on the mistaken notion that intercourse is a highly taxing activity and you need sleep in order to recuperate. When intercourse takes place late at night, it's fine to go to sleep afterward. Among the many functions of sex is facilitating sleep. There is however, no physiological need to sleep after orgasm. The man who routinely rolls over and goes to sleep is cheating both himself and his partner of the warm, intimate, sharing that characterizes afterplay.

For the woman who is nonorgasmic during intercourse, afterplay provides an opportunity for manual stimulation to orgasm. She may find it difficult to request stimulation so he needs to be especially sensitive and responsive to her feelings.

One couple Barry treated for sexual dysfunction—a military officer and his wife—provided an excellent example. The couple had been following a program of pleasuring, making good progress. The wife had been nonorgasmic during intercourse, and he ignored her requests for manual stimulation in afterplay. We talked about her sexual feelings, and he reluctantly agreed the next time he would help her be orgasmic. But after intercourse, he fell asleep. Then, remembering his promise, he roused himself and said in a grumpy voice, "I almost forgot. Is there anything you want me to do?" She became livid. "That's it, I'm leaving you!" She did leave, but came back shortly afterward, and they returned to therapy. He learned to be sensitive to his wife's needs and view her as an equal sexual person. As his attitude changed, she became responsive to his touch and orgasmic both during pleasuring and afterplay.

Another impediment to a man's enjoyment stems from fear that touching or caressing implies a demand for further sexual activity. There is a male physiological phenomenon, the "refractory period," when it is physically impossible to respond to sexual stimulation and regain an erection. This is at least fifteen minutes and can extend to an hour (and much longer for an older man). He feels touching is unnecessary since it cannot lead to anything sexual. He fears if he fails to respond, he will be seen as lacking virility. But if he understands that no further performance is expected, he will relax and enjoy touching, kissing, and holding which makes afterplay such a rewarding experience.

Tenderness and relaxation are the most common responses, but other feelings and activities are possible. As with pleasuring and intercourse, variety, experimentation, and spontaneity are important. A couple may find themselves in a playful, happy mood and express their exuberance by taking a shower together, raiding the refrigerator, or going for a run. As with other phases of sex, optimal satisfaction results when both partners are in touch with their feelings and express them in a free, spontaneous, and mutually sensitive manner.

CLOSING THOUGHTS

When a man is open to sexual variation and experimentation, he increases his pleasure and enhances his relationship. The basic principle of sexual satisfaction is simple. Anything that expands and intensifies a couple's enjoyment is good. Anything that limits or inhibits enjoyment is bad for them (though not necessarily for others). The rest is up to you. Sexuality is yours to make of what you will. Why not make the most of touching, pleasuring, intercourse, and afterplay?

8
LEARNING ABOUT SEXUALITY: THE SINGLE MAN

Before the 1960s, sex among single people was unofficially regulated by the double standard. Unmarried men and women were expected to conform to quite different codes of conduct. For an adolescent boy, intercourse was a goal to be achieved as his rite of passage to manhood. Masculinity and sexuality were closely related. The young man felt overwhelming pressure to prove himself sexually. Virginity was an embarrassment, a mark of shame. No adolescent male over sixteen would admit to being a virgin (although the large majority were in the 1960s—and half still are in the 1990s). The young man who "scored" with the greatest number of women was an object of envy and admiration by his peers.

The adolescent female, on the other hand, was taught her sexuality was a valuable possession to be protected—saved in a hope chest—until it could be bestowed untarnished on a husband (or at least a fiancée). The limits of acceptable female sexual behavior varied from family to family and community to community, but one rule remained constant: unmarried women were not supposed to "go all the way." They were expected to remain virgins until marriage, or to have premarital sex only with the man they planned to marry.

PRESSURE ON WOMEN
The double standard created an interesting dilemma. If young men were expected to be sexually experienced before marriage

while young women were not, with whom were the young men supposed to acquire their experience? The solution depended on the existence of two classes of women—"good girls" and "bad girls." Good girls were the ones who followed society's dictates and remained virginal. Bad girls were the ones who gave in—who had intercourse, thereby "cheapening" themselves. In actuality, this distinction was not strictly maintained. Not every girl who had sex before marriage become "bad." It was only when she acquired a reputation, was known to be "easy," that her social standing was threatened. Interestingly, this was the reverse for males; a young man's reputation for promiscuity enhanced rather than diminished his status.

PRESSURE ON MEN

The double standard allowed greater sexual freedom for single men. Yet, it imposed severe restrictions on male sexual expression. Because "scoring" was such an indispensable sign of masculinity, sex was competitive, performance- and number-oriented. Women were viewed as sexual objects, trophies in the game of sexual conquest. A considerable degree of manipulativeness was condoned so a young man could "make" a woman. He was expected to be false and seductive, to pretend a greater intimacy than he felt—all in the interest of getting her to "come across" and go to bed with him. Male "lines" to convince women to be sexual were the material for jokes and books. They changed with the fads, but the common theme was it was a game, a manipulation.

This persistent pursuit got young men the reputation of "only having one thing on their mind"—sex. In truth, it was not just sexual intercourse that spurred them on; it was the glory of having had sex, the great initiating experience that was so crucial in confirming his manhood. Sex as status, sex as accomplishment—these were the motivations. Genuine sexual feelings played a part, but the quality of the experience was viewed as unimportant. The real emphasis was on competition with his peers. As in poker, bluffing was a legitimate tactic in this sexual game. He would fabricate or exaggerate his exploits in order to advance himself in the eyes of friends. This set the stage for the pattern which extends throughout men's lifespan—brag and "one up," never admit problems or ask questions, be the self-contained sex expert.

Young men were so caught up in the pursuit of sexual conquest that much of the pleasure was lost. Premarital sex was surrounded by societal sanctions and inhibitions so young people, both male and female, were too anxious and ill at ease to enjoy sexuality in anything approaching its full potential. The double standard not only imposed separate codes of behavior on men and women, but made them ill suited as sexual partners. They identified with stereotyped role models—men were expected to be aggressive and women passive. Whole areas of experience, feelings, pleasure, and communication were closed off for each sex. Males were eager for sex, open to sexual experimentation, focused on sexual performance. On the other hand, men did not develop a capacity for tenderness and caring, they were unable to integrate intimate emotions with the physical expression of sex. For males, *sex* meant "intercourse." If there was only affection and pleasuring, the woman had gotten the best of him—he labeled her a "cock teaser." Women were less enthusiastic about sex, less adventurous, and afraid of negative consequences (pregnancy, low self-esteem, censure of family and friends). HIV/AIDS was not a factor in the 1960s. Yet, women were more open to and valued relationships, and had a greater appreciation for affection, sensuality, feelings, and communication.

LEAVING THE DOUBLE STANDARD BEHIND
There have been major changes in our attitudes toward sexuality, with much of this change focused on premarital sex. The double standard is no longer dominant. Women have stepped out of their passive role, they are active and value sexuality. The old sanctions against premarital sex have broken down. It is the norm for single men and women to have intercourse during adolescence and early adulthood. In fact, most sex educators (not to mention parents and ministers) believe the pendulum has swung too far. Over 90 percent of men and 85 percent of women have intercourse before marriage. Two trends are prominent. The first is delaying marriage. The average age for males to marry is 26

(compared to 23 in the 1960s) and for females 24 (compared to 21 in the 1960s). Second, the average age to begin intercourse has decreased to 17 for males (compared to 19 in the 1960s) and 18 for females (compared to 21 in the 1960s). Men and women are involved in premarital sex for longer periods of time and with more partners.

Premarital sexual experience no longer brands a young woman as "bad." In fact, being a virgin can be as much of a burden to a woman as to a man. The double standard is no longer the cultural norm, but continues to have a major influence, interfering with sexual communication and pleasure. There is a real question whether what has replaced the double standard is an improvement. It is not easy to develop an emotionally integrated and healthy approach to premarital sexuality.

The new sexual norms require both men and women to live up to the aggressive, competitive standards that used to apply exclusively to men. There is a danger that women, as well as men, put more importance on performance than pleasure. This was ironically demonstrated when Masters and Johnson published their research on female multiple orgasm. Suddenly a new performance demand came into existence, a new standard against which to measure sexual ability. Women who considered themselves sexually liberated felt inadequate if they were not multiorgasmic (less than one in five adult women are multiorgasmic, and the numbers are lower for adolescent and young adult women)[7]. Female performance anxiety manifested itself in the form of secondary orgasmic dysfunction. There is a troubling increase in women who have been orgasmic and are now nonorgasmic, in part as a result of attempts to become multiorgasmic, have "G" spot orgasms, or whatever is the current faddish performance criterion. How unfortunate it would be if the double standard was replaced by a code of behavior that was coercive—exerting pressure to meet a particular standard of performance—rather than genuinely liberating for both men and women.

PUTTING PREMARITAL SEX IN PERSPECTIVE

Part of the problem is premarital sex has been mistakenly viewed as the paramount sexual issue. Whether premarital sex is forced underground by societal sanctions as it was in the past or celebrated and ballyhooed as it is today, the result is the same: premarital sex is overemphasized at the expense of adult sexuality. Contemporary stereotypes portray sex between single people as glamorous, tantalizing, passionate, and explosive. The emphasis on premarital sex as premarital intercourse downplays the range of sexual expression. Sex as an intimate sharing of pleasure between people who are committed to one another is ignored. Whether operating under the old, repressive double standard or the new, coercive single standard, young people feel pressure to ''prove'' themselves sexually. We ought to cease focusing on questions such as ''Should you or shouldn't you have intercourse?'' and look at premarital sex from the perspective of a person's lifetime involvement with sexuality. Instead of seeing the premarital phase as a time of intense sexual activity—a sexual proving ground—it would be healthier to regard it as an initial explorative foray into the world of adult sexuality, a kind of apprenticeship.

A POSITIVE APPROACH TO PREMARITAL SEXUALITY

An honest, nonmanipulative single standard of premarital sexuality needs to be developed—one that would integrate the stereotypical man's eagerness for sexual expression and the woman's interest in feelings and relationships. Rather than women copying men in being sexually manipulative and exploitative, she would be comfortable and sexually expressive in the context of a respectful, communicative, trusting relationship. In turn, the man would accept sexuality as a means of expressing and sharing intimate feelings and giving and receiving pleasure, rather than a self-centered demand to be satisfied through exploitation. The necessary attitude change is for the young man to see the woman as a sexual person rather than an object. A sexual object can be manipulated, used, and discarded. But if regarded as a sexual friend, a woman becomes someone whose needs, both physical and emotional, are respected. What we are advocating is an honest, trusting and respectful relationship between the sexes. Both men and women must be open to change.

The best time for this learning process to begin is at the outset of a person's sexual career—during the premarital years. A young man who is accustomed to being sexually manipulative, has treated sex partners as objects—as prizes to be acquired, and who has had little practice in communicating honestly finds it difficult to change after he is married. Nor do women automatically blossom sexually when they marry. If premarital learning stressed that a woman was not to engage in sex too freely or enthusiastically, this attitude remains after marriage.

The negative effects of the double standard on women have been emphasized, and rightly so. The woman is discouraged from developing an aware, responsible, affirmative view of her sexuality. This inhibits adult sexual expression. Yet, in the long run it is the male who experiences more negative effects from the double standard. The adult male finds it difficult to integrate emotional feelings and sexual expression into a genuinely intimate relationship. He finds it difficult to view his wife as his intimate partner and sexual friend. Males learn to be sexual outside the context of a caring relationship. The young man functions autonomously, he is able to experience desire, arousal, and orgasm without needing anything from his partner. As he ages, he needs a giving, intimate relationship to function and enjoy sex. His premarital socialization inhibits his ability to ask for, much less value, an intimate, interactive relationship. Nor does it help if both partners are influenced by the new false single standard in which men and women are expected to conform to aggressive, competitive sex roles. This model promotes negative sexual experiences and cynicism about intimate relationships. For the sake of achieving fulfillment in adult life, as well as for present satisfaction, it is important for young men (and women) to have positive guidelines for making decisions about sexuality and relationships.

PARTNER CHOICE

A basic issue is whom to choose as a partner. In the past, the double standard made it clear what was expected. But now that it is acceptable for women to express themselves sexually, new issues have arisen. In our society where the choice of sexual behavior is left largely to the individual, the burden of making decisions which are congruent with your personal value system and situation becomes far greater. We no longer have clear ''dos and don'ts'' to rely on.

The double standard was clear, but wrong. Present premarital standards are confusing and unclear. The premarital standard of ''sex with affection'' sounds reasonable, but is difficult to put into practice. In a sense, we are like children whose mother has given us free run of the cookie jar; the question has suddenly changed from ''How many cookies can I get?'' to ''How many and what kind of cookies do I want?'' Are we obligated to prove the vigor of our appetites by gobbling as many as we can get our hands on? The problem is harder for males because they have been schooled in the doctrine that a real man never turns down a sexual opportunity. It is particularly important for single men to establish guidelines for managing our sexual relationships.

CIRCLES OF INTIMACY

Let's start by examining our interpersonal relationships. If we think about the people whose lives touch ours, it becomes apparent we are involved with people on several levels. These involvements can be categorized according to the degree of intimacy they entail. Human relationships are, of course, highly complex, and any attempt to fit them into categories is arbitrary. Nevertheless, it is worthwhile trying, since by doing so we gain a clarity and perspective on relationships generally, and sexual relationships specifically.

Relationships can be seen as fitting into five categories. We can visualize these categories as a series of concentric circles. The closer to the center, the more intimacy involved; the larger the circle, the less intimacy. As the relationship becomes closer, the degree of trust, caring, and emotional involvement increases, but so does vulnerability to hurt and rejection.

In circle E—the outermost circle—are people whose lives intersect with yours, but about whom you know virtually nothing, sometimes not even their names. This group, whose number is potentially unlimited, might include a clerk, bus driver, receptionist, people you say hello to on the street. Your interaction is purely coincidental and involves no intimacy at all. The next circle, D, contains people with whom you have a degree of contact (an acquaintance), but no real personal involvement—people you see on a regular basis and chat with occasionally. You know their name and some facts about them, but if they were to disappear from your life, you would experience little emotional reaction. At any given time there are a hundred or more acquaintances, and during the course of your lifetime, thousands.

Relationships that involve a degree of intimacy begin with circle C. These are people you think of as friends, with whom you spend time, share feelings, and whose attitude toward you is important. You care about them. If they were to disappear from your life, an emotional gap would be created, although not a devastating one. Circle C friends fade as life circumstances change—you move, complete school, change jobs. You may have five to fifteen level C friends at any given time, and more than a hundred in the course of a lifetime.

Circle B involves quality, close friendships. These people know a great deal about you. You trust them and divulge intimate feelings. The average person may have one to five close friends at any given time and ten to thirty-five during his life. These are people you maintain contact with when your life circumstances change. Circle B friendships are an important, ongoing part of your life. Quality friendships contribute to self-esteem and feelings of belonging in the world. When a close relationship comes to an end, you experience sadness and hurt.

Circle A includes very close, intimate relationships such as a best friend, lover, spouse, or an older adult who serves as a mentor or confidante. These relationships involve deep commitment and emotional intimacy. People in circle A know our innermost thoughts, they share our personal strengths and weaknesses. These are people we trust and care about. We expect them to "be there" for us. When a circle A relationship ends, we are affected profoundly, experiencing a deep sense of loss. An example is a divorce. In one's whole life there are usually no more than four to twenty circle A relationships, and for many men there may be one or two.

We can use this circles of intimacy concept to examine the values that serve as a basis for making decisions about sexual relationships. According to the double standard (which assumed a man should be willing and able to have sex with any woman, anytime, anywhere), a woman from any of the circles would be a potential sexual partner. On the other hand, a woman was expected to have sex only with a man occupying circle A—her husband or fiancée. The double standard required a man to utilize deception and manipulation to convince a potential partner his feelings went much deeper than they really did, his level of caring and emotional involvement approached circle B or A.

This is poor preparation for a mature intimate relationship. Be honest and clear about which circle of intimacy a woman who attracts you occupies. This does not necessarily mean you can only have sex with women from circles A and B. It does mean you should not enter into a sexual encounter under false pretenses. For example, it is acceptable for a man and woman whose degree of connection placed them in circle D to be sexual, provided both knew where they stood and were responsible about contraception and safer sex. If, on the other hand, the woman was dissatisfied with a circle D relationship and wished for a degree of intimacy characterized by circle B, it would be unacceptable to pretend such a relationship existed in order to have sex with her. This circles of intimacy concept is equally applicable to women, and could be useful in moving us closer to a responsible single standard of premarital sexual expression. This would provide a healthier basis for adult sexual functioning for men and women alike.

There is nothing inherently wrong with casual sex, so long as the participants have no illusions and practice safer sex in terms of contraception and STDs/HIV. A guideline is if a couple can't talk about contraception and STDs/HIV, they have no business having sex. Sex is more psychologically satisfying when a degree of intimacy exists between the partners. It is easier in an intimate, trusting relationship to be honest about your sexual feelings and preferences, which increases sexual satisfaction.

Assuming you want to enhance the quality of your sex life, you would do well to limit your partners to women from circle C or closer. If you see the woman as a sexual friend you are more likely to communicate about contraception and STDs/HIV. Friends treat each other well. They do not cause problems and hurt.

Using the circles of intimacy concept to plan and order your sex life may at first seem a strange idea. People think sex should be a spontaneous occurrence and planning sexual activity makes it less intense. Actually, planning makes real spontaneity possible and helps avoid problems—as well as increase feelings of comfort and confidence. Sexuality is an integral part of you as a person. Sexuality can enhance your life and relationship rather than cause difficulties and pain.

FIRST INTERCOURSE

Nowhere is planning more needed—yet nowhere is it more avoided—than in first intercourse. Because losing his virginity is so significant, whether it occurs at age fifteen or thirty-five, first intercourse would ideally be planned, adequate contraceptive measures utilized, a condom used to protect against STDs/ HIV, and sex would be enjoyable and satisfying. The experience would be enhanced if the couple was comfortable communicating and had engaged in pleasuring at least once or twice before attempting intercourse. This crucial first experience should be seen not as a performance but as a choiceful event arising from communication, desire, and planning.

Unfortunately, few (if any) men undergo their sexual initiation in such ideal circumstances. Typically, first intercourse is characterized by intense anxiety based partly on fear of failure and partly on fear of being caught. Less than half of first-time couples use effective contraception. The contraceptive device used most frequently is the condom, put on in a hurried, clumsy manner. Since first intercourse is a time of high anxiety, high excitement, and low skill, it is surprising when it goes well. About 25 percent of males experience failure at first intercourse because they ejaculate before the penis enters the vagina, can't get an erection, or lose their erection. The great majority of men ejaculate quickly during first intercourse. It is important not to overreact to an unsuccessful or disappointing first experience. Sexual satisfaction requires cooperation, feedback and practice. Sex improves with time and practice. The man is not a sexual machine who must function flawlessly whenever the button of sexual stimulation is pressed.

PREMARITAL SEXUALITY AS A LEARNING EXPERIENCE

If a young man is able to think of premarital sex not as a "proving ground" but as a learning opportunity, a time of apprenticeship for the long period of mature sexuality to come, the pressure will be diminished. The less you think of sex as a performance and the more you think of it as a learning and enhancing experience, the more enjoyable it will be. Once we accustom ourselves to the fact that we are at a learning stage and are not alone in this, we become accepting of our uncertainties and mistakes. We benefit from these early experiences in ways that promote adult sexual functioning. There is a joy to learning a new skill, and sex is no exception.

There is a feeling of satisfaction in knowing that, from one relationship to the next, you are learning to confront hang-ups, communicate more effectively, make love more sensitively and skillfully, and treat your partner as a sexual friend. Some sexual relationships are mistakes that cause pain and leave bad feelings. These also serve as learning experiences. The value of premarital sex is not in proving yourself a sexual superman, but feeling you are growing as a sexual person. You are learning to make sexuality a positive force in your life, integrating sexuality with your emotions and relationships.

The percentage of men who succeed in making such an adjustment is still not great, but there are enough to hope that comfortable, pleasurable, and learning-oriented premarital sexuality is the wave of the future (for both men and women).

Jon

Jon is an example of a single man who is learning about himself, women, sexuality, and relationships. A twenty-four-year-old graduate student who works as a trainee for a communications company, Jon enjoys his job and is pleased with his sexual life and relationships. He did not have intercourse until nineteen and was concerned he was lagging behind his friends, but gave up these fears when he became sexually active. Most of his affairs involve some level of intimacy. He had four sex partners in about the same number of years. Jon felt little pressure to "score" with a greater number of women merely to achieve prestige

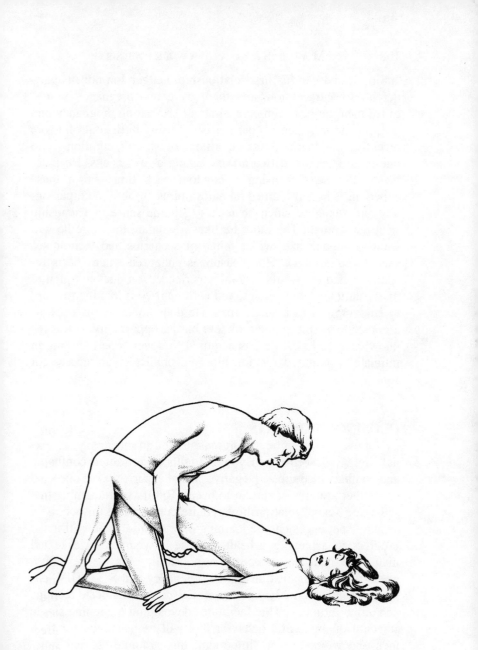

Pleasuring and intercourse are complementary ways of expressing sexual feelings.

among friends. In his first relationship, neither Jon nor his partner used contraception, and there were two pregnancy scares. Since then, he has been careful about preventing pregnancy and uses a condom when his partner is not using birth control. More recently, Jon has had sexual affairs of shorter duration—two one-night stands and two affairs lasting a few weeks. He practiced safer sex by using a condom each time. From these experiences he has learned he enjoys himself more, both personally and sexually, when he feels a genuine sense of friendship with the woman. The more he likes a woman, the more he will want to engage in a wider range of scenarios and techniques, such as cunnilingus. His pleasure is enhanced when she is responsive and enjoys the sexual experience. Jon does not plan to marry until his late twenties, and until married is looking forward to enjoying sex as a single man. He does not view marriage as a comedown from premarital sex, but an opportunity to use the knowledge and skill he has acquired to develop and sustain an intimate, committed relationship. We predict great success for Jon.

CLOSING THOUGHTS

Not everyone can be as fortunate as Jon in managing his sexual life. Adolescence and young adulthood are often confusing and conflict-filled times. Negative sexual experiences of one kind or another are almost certain to occur. But if you remember that satisfying sexual relationships require comfort and unsuccessful sexual experiences can be learning opportunities, you will make progress in achieving a healthy sense of yourself as a sexual man. The man, in accepting responsibility for his sexuality, needs to guard against unwanted pregnancy and STDs/HIV, enjoy experimentation, be open to eroticism, communicate feelings and value intimacy. This facilitates developing a genuine single standard of premarital behavior that will be beneficial for both men and women. More important, this promotes sexual functioning and satisfaction throughout life.

9

MARRIAGE: CHOOSING THE INTIMATE BOND

Sadie Hawkins Day was a holiday celebrated by the citizens of Dogpatch, the backwoods community portrayed in the classic comic strip, "Li'l Abner." During Sadie Hawkins Day, it was open season on males. Any woman who managed to run down, corner, and trap a single man had the right to claim him as her spouse. The holiday was enormously popular with the women of Dogpatch. But to the men, Sadie Hawkins Day was a time of pure terror, when each member of Dogpatch's bachelor population exercised his utmost talents of evasion to avoid "a fate worse'n death."

What makes Sadie Hawkins Day so funny is its devastatingly accurate caricature of traditional male attitudes toward marriage. We see ourselves entering into marriage under protest. The rewards of marriage—closeness, intimacy, security—are supposed to matter only to women. Men value freedom, good times, and sexual variety. Women are involved in a continual effort to ensnare men into marriage, to deprive them of their freedom, and turn them into tame, obedient husbands. How close we still are to the Sadie Hawkins Day mentality can be seen from the way we respond to news of a friend's marital plans. The language is analogous to descriptions of defeat in battle. "Another good man gone," or "Another man bites the dust." We jokingly offer our condolences.

The contrast between male and female attitudes toward marriage can be seen in the celebrations that precede the wedding ceremony. The bridal shower happily looks forward to the married state. The bachelor party, which features drunkenness and salaciousness, is a last look backward at the joys of single life and unencumbered sex.

THE REAL MALE ATTITUDE TOWARD MARRIAGE

But isn't there a discrepancy? Statistics show over 90 percent of men marry. Marriage is neither going out of style nor is it a dying institution. Even with a greatly heightened divorce rate, it is men who enter into second marriages more often and more quickly than women. If we are really engaged in a battle against the efforts of marriage-minded women to enslave us, then we must be extremely ineffectual warriors. Either that or there is a good deal of hypocrisy in our attitude.

The second explanation is correct. It isn't only women who desire the intimacy and security marriage is designed to provide. These are human needs, not just female ones. Marriage holds the promise of an emotional and sexual bond that is deeper, more secure and more satisfying than possible in any other relationship. Women respond to this promise wholeheartedly because they have learned from childhood to think of marriage as a desirable goal. Men feel they must hold back because marriage does not coincide with the macho ideal. He desires the rewards marriage offers, but, for the sake of appearances, represents himself as another Sadie Hawkins Day casualty.

The trouble with this attitude is a man who pretends to enter the married state under duress feels that merely consenting to marriage is all that should be required. Men believe they don't need to bring emotional energy or personal commitment to marriage. For a woman, marriage is supposed to be everything, the very basis of her life (this is an unhealthy extreme—marriage should be one-quarter, at the most one-third, of self-esteem for a man or woman). The traditional view was marriage is merely one of several obligations a man undertakes, and not the most important. Many men feel marriage is a matter of fulfilling set duties, and completing these puts him above criticism. This attitude is typified by a cartoon in which a husband and wife are seated in their living room. The man glances over his newspaper with a look of consternation and says: "Of course I love you— that's my job." Men settle for minimally involving marriages.

A marriage conducted in this spirit will become unsatisfying.

A man undertakes the responsibilities of marriage in the same way he undertakes the responsibilities of his business, but there the resemblance between the two institutions ends. A company is able to survive if employees do their jobs in an uninspired, routine way. American marriages do not have the extensive family and community support available in cultures such as Ireland or India. American marriages require a quality relationship to survive and thrive. There are no stockholders in a marriage, no federal subsidies, no way of borrowing emotional capital. The marital bond of respect, trust, and intimacy must be valued and reinforced by the couple. Entropy, the tendency of a system to break down if left to itself, gradually subverts the marital bond. A love that isn't growing is dying. If the man wants a satisfying and secure marriage he has to invest himself in his intimate relationship.

Empirical research supports the idea that a good marriage is a major contributor to psychological well-being for both men and women. Women value and enjoy their marriages more, which is paradoxical because, contrary to popular myths, men need marriage more than women. Compared to single or divorced men, married men function better in terms of physical health, emotional well-being and sexual frequency and satisfaction.

NEGATIVE REASONS TO MARRY

Because marriage is a major life choice, it is foolish and self-defeating to enter into it with anything less than readiness to work toward making it successful. True, there is great pressure to marry in our society. After age 35, unmarried people are looked upon as being a bit strange, and single men are suspected of being gay. Nevertheless, you can resist social pressure. Marriage is one of a number of options (staying single, cohabitation, serious monogamous affairs). Marry only if you decide that person fits your needs and life values, and the marriage will be viable and satisfying.

The first step in assessing whether you are marrying for the right reasons is to determine whether you are choosing marriage for its own sake or to escape from something else. For instance, a man may marry to avoid the pressures of dating or loneliness.

He may see marriage as the only way to escape an abusive or stifling family situation. He allows parental or peer pressure to force him to marry. One of the worst reasons to marry is an attempt to cover up a real or suspected homosexual orientation. In such situations, marriage is not a positive choice but an avoidance of dealing with an issue (a strategy which won't work).

Be extremely suspicious of your motives when a course of action appears to be "the only way out." When people seek marriage because it is "time to settle down," they do not give the time and attention to choose a compatible spouse. He's so anxious to marry that he ends up with whoever happens to be convenient or available. If this is how the partner is chosen, the level of respect and caring is lowered. The man discovers his interests and values are so different than his wife's that they can't develop a viable life together. It compounds the difficulty any two people have in adjusting to each other's idiosyncrasies and handling the hassles and confusions of sharing everyday life. Marriage is something to positively choose, not back into.

For some men, marriage is a symbol of being an independent, mature adult. However, men who marry before age twenty-one have a very high divorce rate. You need to establish your own identity and goals before marrying. Postponing marriage until the early or mid-twenties is a healthier decision.

An unplanned pregnancy is a very poor reason to marry. Marrying the woman you have gotten pregnant may seem like the right thing to do, and such an action may have been laudable at a time when the stigma of giving birth to an illegitimate child was high. Today it is a far greater kindness to consider marriage as a choice in and of itself, rather than a way of avoiding an abortion or giving up a child for adoption. Don't go to the other extreme and automatically eliminate marriage as a solution to an unplanned pregnancy. The fact is one of four brides is pregnant at the time of marriage or already has a child. These couples can create a viable marital bond—especially those who were already planning to marry and moved up the date because of the pregnancy.

Just as marrying the pregnant woman can be a gallant but unrealistic resolution, marrying a man to reform him is its equally foolish female counterpart. The woman who marries a man with a drinking or gambling problem, who can't hold a job, has multiple affairs, or can't make emotional commitments, thinking that her good influence will cause him to reform, is being unrealistic. It is the man's responsibility to change his life. Dealing with those problems is the job of individual therapy, not marriage. No matter how well intentioned a wife may be, it is unlikely she will be able to reform him. Nor is it her role to do so. A man who is motivated to change and assumes responsibility for change greatly benefits from a helpful, supportive spouse. But she can't do it for him; he has to change for himself with her help. The man has to be more committed to his change process than the woman. One sign of a good marriage is it brings out the best in each person.

POSITIVE REASONS TO MARRY

So much for poor reasons. What are the positive reasons to marry? Marriage provides benefits it would be difficult to realize in any other relationship. A good marriage offers emotional intimacy, vital sexuality, sense of connection, stability, and a life companion. Sharing the highs as well as everyday events, a married couple has an opportunity to develop a caring, connected life. A man's need to feel loved, respected, and secure and to love and care for another person is satisfied better through marriage than any other relationship. Of course, there can be a dark side to marriage. Married couples fall into the traps of boredom and psychological suffocation. He surrenders his individuality and halts personal growth. The insights into one another's character that marriage offers can be used to wound rather than help. This is caused by an insufficiently thought-out marriage decision, a lack of commitment, an inability to address and resolve conflicts, or a lack of respect for the spouse or marriage. The security and intimacy of a good marriage is one of the best experiences life can offer, but both people have to make the psychological investment and commitment.

CHOOSING A SPOUSE

Just as there are positive and negative reasons for getting married, there are healthy and unhealthy ways of choosing a mate. Perhaps the single most important element is respect—respect for the person and respect for the way you are as a couple. With your marital partner, you choose a life course—whether to have children and how many, where and how to live, the work you do and how it is integrated into your life, your values. After the glow of romantic love has worn off (which lasts one or two years at the most), the marital bond of respect, trust, and intimacy must be valued and strengthened.

A very important prerequisite is your ability to communicate. Communication involves a capacity and willingness to share important aspects of your lives and personalities, not just those that make you look good. A marriage partner is someone with whom you can talk about fears and disappointments as well as hopes and dreams. Allowing your partner to know vulnerable areas as well as strengths builds intimacy. Revealing weaknesses—feelings of uncertainty and inadequacy or sadness and depression—is one of the hardest things for a man to do. Males learn from an early age they must always be, or appear to be, in control. The myth is women admire "the strong, silent type." Certainly, strength is an admirable quality in any human being, male or female. But no sensible person would expect a partner to be strong on all occasions. The spouse must be willing to accept you as you are rather than what she wants you to be. Especially important is accepting vulnerabilities and weaknesses without putting you down.

Involvement needs to be reciprocal. The spouse should not take the role of therapist or confessor. She is honest and open about her thoughts and feelings, both positive and negative. Effective communication includes the inevitable dissatisfactions and disagreements that occur in any marriage. There is strong empirical support for the critical importance of being able to deal with and resolve conflicts. Just as important, couples need to be able to enjoy time and activities together, to share good feelings. Friends who are supportive of you as people and your marriage are a helpful resource.

The first two years of marriage are crucial in developing a couple style which is comfortable and functional for both people. Contrary to the cultural myth that all happy marriages are similar with the more intimacy the better, empirical research has identified four viable marital styles. These are:

1. Complementary couples: Each spouse identifies his/her do-

main of influence, this role is acknowledged and respected by the partner, there are moderate amounts of intimacy with room for individual prerogatives. This is the most common marital style.

2. Conflict-minimizing couples: This is the most predictable and stable marital model where each spouse has his/her domain, usually established along traditional male-female roles. They value marital security. The danger is too little intimacy and not enough sharing of activities and feelings.

3. Best friend couple: This model involves the most amount of intimacy and closeness and is viewed as the ideal. The danger is losing one's individuality and feeling bitter or disappointed if the marriage does not live up to its promise.

4. Emotionally expressive couple: This is the most emotionally vital, but also the most unstable couple style. There are high degrees of intimacy, but also high degrees of anger and conflict. The key is not to allow conflicts to degenerate into criticalness and alienation.

Of course, no couple is a "pure" type, but one task in choosing a partner and developing a couple style is to reach clear understandings. For example, one partner wanting an emotionally expressive marriage and the other wanting a conflict minimizing marriage results in a fatally flawed relationship.

During the first two years of married life couples increase sensitivity to one another's moods and preferences, but people aren't mind readers. Communication remains extremely important. When joys and sorrows are not shared and instead suppressed, the couple is neither able to feel satisfaction nor identify and work on problem areas. Choosing a marital partner you can trust and talk to, sharing feelings and confronting conflicts, is crucial.

How important is sexual attraction and functioning in choosing a spouse? Paradoxically, sexual problems are a reason to carefully assess whether the marriage is viable, but good sex is not predictive of a healthy marriage or even predictive of marital sex. In fact, couples who report romantic love with intense and passionate premarital sex are more likely to become disappointed and develop a sexual dysfunction. There are three potential sexual poisons. The first is she (or you) withholds a sexual secret (about a previous marriage, arrest for sex crime, sexual orientation issue, sexual trauma, having fathered a child). A second is a lack of sexual desire for partner (seen as best friend, but no sexual attraction). A third is if there is a sexual dysfunction and the partner is not willing to deal with it. At its core, marriage is a respectful, trusting friendship. Sex should not be a deciding factor in marital choice.

Another important guideline is to choose someone whose interests and values are compatible. If they share interests, the couple will be more likely to spend enjoyable time together. Conflicts over values create strains. Of course, interests and values need not all coincide, It's helpful to have activities and interests not shared with your spouse. This allows you to maintain individuality. Balancing autonomy and coupleness is an ongoing challenge. The strongest marriages are those in which there are both shared and separate areas of interest, where the partners have much in common, yet each brings something unique to the marriage. Although people talk about how opposites attract, the empirical data are clear—people from similar backgrounds, interests, and values have more stable and satisfying marriages.

Before a couple decide to marry, they should discuss realistically the major issues that will confront them. Questions to focus on are: Will there be children, and if so, when? How will the couple manage and spend money, and what are their financial priorities? Where will they live? What roles will each spouse take with regard to careers, housekeeping, and child rearing? How important is sexuality? Will the couple maintain fidelity or can certain types of extramarital affairs be tolerated? How committed is each partner to making this a satisfying and stable marriage? What sort of contact will they have with extended family? These core issues need to be dealt with before marriage, at least developing realistic understandings and awareness of sensitive issues.

There is a strong tendency for a couple anticipating marriage to minimize difficulties. This is especially true of younger couples who feel that by being romantic and insisting love will solve all problems, they can preserve the idealistic glow. Building a marriage on romantic love is like building a home on sand—it will quickly erode. For a marriage to succeed you need communication, problem-solving, and realistic planning. Problem-solving and planning are compatible with mature love, but antithetical to romantic love.

THE PROCESS OF A SUCCESSFUL MARRIAGE

Functioning as a married person is, like other forms of behavior, something we learn. It helps to have a good role model. If one or both partners was raised by parents who were happily married, a healthy marital relationship is the norm. If you have not had such good fortune, adopt the opposite strategy and try to learn from the weaknesses of your parents. This couple must work harder and more consciously to achieve a successful marriage.

Both Emily and Barry fit the latter category. Our parents' marriages were stressful and unhappy. We were strongly committed to having a successful marriage. During the first two years we consciously built a bond of respect, trust and intimacy. We were so pleased with our initial success, we became complacent. We were at a plateau, and in danger of stagnating. We made the decision to work at enhancing our relationship. This proved easier for Emily than Barry. Like most men, Barry had a lower expectation of marriage. Communicating effectively, being affectionate, and thinking as a couple rather than as a single person who happened to be married required conscious effort. Barry has found the effort worthwhile, both for him as a man and for us as a couple. Several times since we've gone through similar periods of reassessment and refocusing, which can be of immense value in any marriage. We've been married 30 years, yet realize marriage can't rest on its laurels. Marriage is like a garden; it requires a solid foundation, but also needs to be consistently tended, weeded, watered and replanted. If you want it to continue to flower, devote time and psychological energy to your marriage.

Many couples think about marriage only when the relationship is in trouble—the "wait for a crisis" approach. If a marriage is valued, then it is worthwhile to make it better, to increase the dividends it produces. It is a lot easier and more fun to make a good marriage better than lift a bad one off the rocks. Unfortunately, many couples do not try to change their marriages or go for counseling until serious problems have arisen and anger, resentment, blaming and hopelessness have accumulated. The old adage about an ounce of prevention being better than a pound of cure is especially true of marriage.

SEX IN AN ONGOING MARRIAGE

So far we have said little about the role of sex in marriage. Obviously, it has a very important place, but only by first viewing marriage in its larger context can we appreciate marital sex. Our culture offers confusing messages about the importance of marital sex. One viewpoint is sex forms a bedrock—if sex is good, everything else will be good. By the same token, if trouble appears, the cause can be traced to poor sex. Another viewpoint is that sex is of minor importance, the primary element is love. If the relationship is loving, sex doesn't matter.

These extreme attitudes are wrong. Sex serves a number of functions in marriage. Most important, it helps to create and reinforce feelings of intimacy. Sex provides a shared pleasure, an affirmation of you as a person and couple. Sex serves as a tension reducer, a refuge from the hassles of bills, children, and stresses of everyday life. Sex is not the primary measure of marriage. It is quite possible for a couple to have a good sexual relationship and yet have serious problems that can destroy the marriage.

Sex is best seen as one aspect of a couple's expression of intimacy. It is not something separate, it's integral to their relationship. A favorite saying among therapists is when sex is good it constitutes 15 to 20 percent of the marriage, energizing the marital bond. When sex is dysfunctional or nonexistent it plays an inordinately powerful role, up to 75 percent, draining the marriage of positive feelings. It is possible for a couple to be emotionally compatible and yet have an unsatisfactory sex life, but it is not possible for them to remain in such a situation indefinitely, at least not without diminishing their relationship or putting it in jeopardy. If a couple is committed to making their marriage successful and getting as much joy and fulfillment as possible, they will not be satisfied with dysfunctional sex. They can work together to develop a comfortable, pleasurable, and functional couple sexual style.

Closeness and sharing is very important for a couple's sexual life. Feeling loved and loving facilitates sexual desire. Many men ignore this; they feel sex is unrelated to anything else. In fact, closeness and affection outside the bedroom is of great importance to sexual vitality. When a husband shows he cares by expressing his hopes and fears, sharing household tasks, calling during the day just to say hello, or planning a special couple evening, he creates intimate feelings which facilitate sexual desire. Intercourse is only one method of sharing sexual pleasure. In the larger context of marriage, sexuality is but one way to express intimacy.

This point is especially important for men who feel each touch must culminate in intercourse. This attitude, common to a surprising number of men, is an outgrowth of the tendency to compartmentalize sex, to see it as a specific act which must be played out according to an unvarying performance script. When the expectation of intercourse is attached to every hug, kiss, and caress, the woman begins to avoid affection. She feels if she's not prepared to go all the way, it is best not to start. Paradoxically, this attitude of "intercourse or nothing" is responsible for reducing intercourse frequency. When partners do not feel free to express their affection both inside and outside the bedroom without the demand of intercourse, they lose in all ways. The level of touching and sensuality is reduced and they have less frequent intercourse. Touching both inside and outside the bedroom, with no expectation that all touching ends in intercourse, promotes affection, sensuality, eroticism and intercourse.

SEXUAL COMMUNICATION

Communication in the couple's daily interaction is clearly related to their sexual relationship. Partners who speak freely on a wide variety of subjects and are able to discuss negative as well as positive feelings are better prepared for the intimate communication which is necessary for healthy sexual functioning. Each person has the right to let the spouse know whether a particular touch is pleasurable or not. No matter how good a lover your partner may be, there is no way she can know what turns you on unless you provide feedback. Men feel they should know how to be good lovers and satisfy their wives without her requests or guidance. But, of course, the theme of this book is men *do* need to learn about sexuality (their own and their spouse's) in order to realize its potential. Both the man and woman have to communicate sexual likes and dislikes if they are to maintain a vital sexual relationship.

Many couples report sex was best premaritally. Newness, excitement, illicitness and frequency carried the sex. For sex to remain good, the couple have to communicate and create quality sexual scenarios. It takes couples at least six months to develop a functional and satisfying sexual style.

If you doubt this is true, try the following test. Can you name all the parts of your partner's body she enjoys having stimulated (for example, breasts, lips, ears, shoulders, thighs, labia, clitoris)? What sort of stimulation does she like (heavy, light, tickling, rubbing, kissing, licking, stroking)? Does she prefer single or multiple stimulation? What pleasuring scenarios are most arousing for her? Do you know her two favorite intercourse positions? Does she like multiple stimulation during intercourse? What is her favorite manner of experiencing afterplay/ afterglow? If you feel unsure about any of the answers, there are things you can learn. To increase awareness, experiment with different pleasuring scenarios and provide feedback, either verbal or nonverbal. Exploration increases knowledge of each other's bodies and sexual preferences. It not only makes you better sex partners, but can be an intimate and adventurous couple experience. Remain open and aware as the marriage progresses. People's sexual preferences change as they discover new areas of sensitivity and learn to experience their bodies in new ways. Communicate these changes and stay in touch sexually.

It cannot be emphasized too strongly that sexual communication is a two-way street. Just as your commitment to the success of the marriage obligates you to be receptive to her signals, so it is your responsibility to communicate your preferences. Sex is a pleasurable activity, and pleasure means asking for what you want. Renunciation and self-sacrifice have no role in marital sexuality.

The first step is knowing what you want. Exploration on your own as well as with your partner can increase awareness. The second step is making these preferences known. This increases your chances of getting what you want as well as diminishes

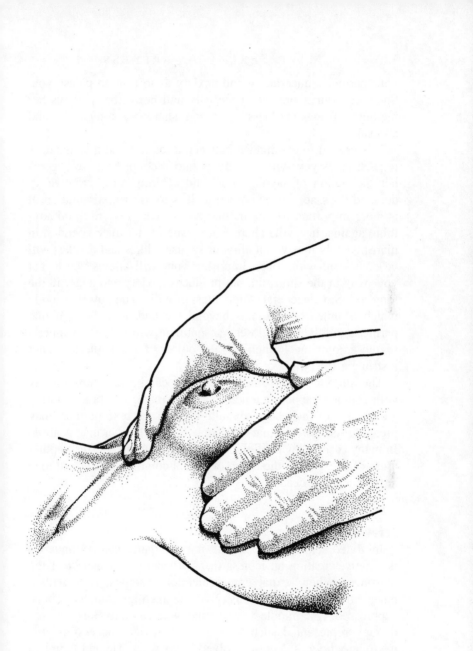

Affectionate, sensual, and erotic touching are integral to the sexual communication process.

your partner's uncertainty and anxiety as to how to please you. Showing your appreciation verbally and nonverbally allays her feelings of awkwardness. She can share your pleasure and arousal.

It is crucial to distinguish between a request and a demand. A request takes your wife's feelings into account because it gives her the option of saying "no" and offering an alternative. A demand does not. As important as it is to ask for stimulation, it is more important for the partner not to feel pressure to do anything against her will. There is no place for intimate coercion in marriage. Obviously, not all your spouse's likes and dislikes will be consistent with yours. Imposing your will allows you to get your way in the short run, but produces anxiety and anger in the long run. Sex degenerates into a test of wills. The power struggle which is unleashed extends beyond the bedroom. Even if one partner capitulates, the loser's resentment will sour the winner's sexual enjoyment. Remember, the object of sex is pleasure, not a struggle for power or control.

The importance of sexual connection can be seen most clearly with couples trapped in a nonsexual marriage. The fault is rarely a total lack of interest in sex, although one or both partners may pretend it is. Nor is it that the couple find each other unappealing. In many cases, they continue to remain on amiable terms in other areas of life. It is in the realm of sexual communication that they have reached a dead end.

Jerry and Fran

Inhibited sexual desire and sexual avoidance can continue indefinitely, creating an iciness that pervades every aspect of the marriage. When sexual communication resumes, it is with a bang, attesting to the intensity of the feelings that have been suppressed. One middle-years couple who came to Barry for sex therapy represented such a case. Jerry was a successful businessman who was deeply involved in his work. He and Fran had not had intercourse for thirteen years and not touched affectionately for eight years. Fran wanted a divorce, but Jerry objected, claiming it would damage his professional image and he valued the stability and companionship of the marriage. They agreed to try sex therapy.

We talked about sexual communication and the value of non-demand touching. Barry suggested they begin with a nongenital pleasuring exercise. Neither seemed enthusiastic, but they promised to try.

When they appeared for the next session, Barry was surprised to see Jerry with a bandage over his right eye that did not completely cover a hideous, purple bruise. When asked what happened, they glanced sheepishly at one another, then, not without a degree of humor, began to tell their story. They had begun the first pleasuring session by having a drink. The exercise suggests holding hands, but when Jerry reached for Fran's hand she jerked it away, saying they had not held hands for years and it was stupid to start now. They finished their drinks and went on to the next step, which was to take a shower together. Fran entered the shower first. Then Jerry entered, and while reaching for the soap, inadvertently brushed against her shoulder. This triggered unexpressed hurt and anger in Fran, for impulsively she turned and rammed her knee into his groin, pushed him out of the shower, then grabbed his hair and smashed his head against the side of the tub.

After Fran had gotten over her fury and begun to apologize, and after Jerry recovered from his initial pain, their reaction was a shocked realization of how physically and sexually alienated they had been. They understood for the first time the strength of the emotions that had been bottled up. Both felt strongly motivated to continue therapy and build a touching and erotic connection. Their ability to communicate improved dramatically. They made rapid progress and successfully revitalized their sexual relationship.

SEX IN ONGOING MARRIAGES

Few marriages suffer from a sexual communication problem as severe as Jerry and Fran's, but most marriages could profit from making communication both in and out of the bedroom sensitive and explicit. Communication, openness, playfulness, and a willingness to experiment are key elements in keeping marital sex from becoming boring and routine. This is a joint responsibility. Each spouse is responsible to communicate his or her emotions, thoughts, feelings, and preferences, as well as be

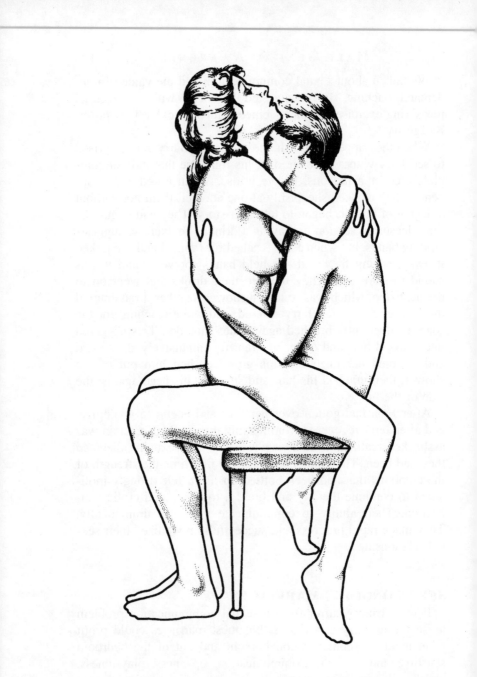

One of many creative positions for intercourse. Such creativity leads to savoring and prolonging the experience rather than a frenzied rush to orgasm.

receptive to the partner's. Each can contribute to the variety and spontaneity of affectionate, sensual, and erotic touching.

This includes refusing to fall into the rut of always using one sexual scenario. It means experimenting with different styles of intercourse—serious, playful, quiet, intense, "quickie," or prolonged and romantic. It means being open to both intentional, planned sexual dates and spontaneous sex. Experiment with making love at different times of day rather than adhering to the arbitrary dictum that the time for intercourse is just before sleep. Try sex in places besides the bedroom—on the living room sofa, on the rug, in the guest bedroom, in front of the fireplace. It means having the forethought to add creative touches to lovemaking such as music, incense, lotions, candles, or an after sex bottle of chilled champagne. Such variations and innovations are not extraneous trappings, they're part of lovemaking. Creative sexual play enhances intimacy and marital sexuality.

CLOSING THOUGHTS

Ideally a man would marry because he wants to, not because he should. He would enter marriage willingly and with his eyes open, not as the victim of Sadie Hawkins Day pressure. He would have positive, realistic expectations of marriage, not a romantic idealism or a cynical settling for a marginal marriage. Every couple goes through negative experiences that need to be dealt with. Facing conflicts with confidence that you can resolve them is a major marital resource. A good marriage requires commitment, energy, and communication. The man owes it to himself (and his spouse) to exert every effort to make his marriage succeed—not out of consideration for marriage in the abstract, but because a good marriage is a source of pleasure, intimacy and security. A successful marriage is well worth the thought, work, and energy needed to make it that way.

10

BRIDGES TO SEXUAL DESIRE, FANTASIES, AND ORAL SEX

Twenty-year-old men learn about sex as easy, automatic, and autonomous. Masculinity and sexuality are strongly associated so it is quite rare for young males to experience inhibited sexual desire. However, by early or mid-thirties the pattern of easy, automatic sex is weaker. Intimate, interactive sex becomes the pattern by the forties. Why wait until your 40s or you experience a sexual dysfunction? Appreciating intimate, interactive sex in your twenties is the best way to enhance sexual pleasure and prevent sexual problems.

This chapter will focus on three strategies—bridges to sexual desire, fantasy and oral sex—to enhance satisfaction. To maintain a vital sexuality the prescription is intimacy, pleasuring, and eroticism.

Sexual desire is the core of sexuality, especially in an intimate relationship. The key components in sexual desire are anticipation and feeling you deserve pleasure. Be aware of the positive functions sexuality can play for you individually and as a couple. You are responsible for your sexuality and deserve to express sexuality so it enhances your self-esteem, intimate relationship, and life. To maintain desire, value the positive functions of sexuality: a shared pleasure, to reinforce and deepen intimacy, and a tension reducer to deal with the hassles of life and a relationship.

Desire problems are more common among women than men. That's because masculinity and sexuality are closely associated and arousal is easy—the best example being spontaneous erections. This changes over time. The significant change in a man's

126

sexual response is it's no longer autonomous—he doesn't get fast, predictable, spontaneous erections. Male response becomes more like female responsivity—both need intimacy and stimulation. Men who accept and enjoy flexible, variable sexuality will maintain sexual desire. Her involvement and arousal increases his desire and arousal. Men who long for the "good old days" and become distracted by performance fears set themselves up for inhibited sexual desire.

BUILDING SEXUAL BRIDGES

There are a range of sexual experiences and a variety of ways to initiate sexual interaction. Sexuality is a one-two combination: personal responsibility and couple intimacy. Each person is responsible for his sexuality, including desire. Intimate sexuality is about initiating, sharing, facilitating, and encouraging. It's not only normal, but preferable, for each partner to have his/her bridges for desire. Having a multitude of ways to anticipate and initiate sexual experiences ensures desire will remain vital. It is healthy for the man and couple to have a variety of ways to share intimacy and pleasure. Choice, rather than obligation, enhances sexual desire. When sex degenerates into "are we going to have intercourse or not?" the couple are in trouble. When the man demands intercourse and the woman avoids pressure and coercion, the result is a sexual power struggle which subverts desire.

Desire is the core of couple sexuality. The optimal prescription for sexual desire is anticipation, an emotionally intimate relationship, nondemand pleasuring, erotic scenarios and techniques, sharing orgasm, feeling emotionally bonded and satisfied, and maintaining a regular rhythm of sexual activities. Anticipation is the central ingredient. Anticipation cannot be willed, forced, or coerced, but can be facilitated and nurtured. Although our culture celebrates romantic, spontaneous, intense, nonverbal sexual initiations, you also need to be open to "intentional, planned sexual dates." It can be fun to set aside time, think about, and anticipate being sexual. Sex becomes relegated to late at night. Being alive, awake, and aware facilitates anticipation. Many men (and couples) prefer sex in the morning, a "nooner," before or after a nap, or early evening sex when there's more energy. Late at night after a stressful day, your testosterone level is reduced by one quarter to one third.

Another bridge to sexual desire is the freedom to make requests, especially for special turn-ons. Ten minutes of foreplay, five minutes of intercourse, and thirty seconds of afterplay does not promote anticipation. Sexual scenarios and turn-ons include being sexual in the shower, playing out a fantasy scenario, using oral sex to build arousal, sexy clothing, mixing sex with wine and gourmet food, using candles and music for special effects.

Intimacy is a major bridge for sexual desire. The most satisfying sex integrates intimacy with eroticism. Traditional sexual socialization taught men to value eroticism and women to value intimacy. Sexual desire is robust when each partner values intimacy, pleasure, and eroticism. Not valuing intimacy is a male trap. Men under 30 need little from the partner to feel desire, arousal, and orgasm. This does not serve the man well, especially in marriage. If sexual desire is to remain vital, he needs to appreciate intimate, interactive sexuality. An involved, aroused partner is the major aphrodisiac. Desire is inhibited by self-consciousness, competitiveness, and performance orientation. Desire is enhanced by intimacy, giving and receiving erotic stimulation, and a pleasure orientation.

Anticipating a sexual scenario is a powerful bridge for desire. Rather than waiting for desire to occur "naturally" or hoping for a spontaneous erection, use sexual fantasies, develop sexual scenarios, and utilize erotic techniques to facilitate desire. For example, if you have a sexual daydream or see an attractive person in a store, allow that erotic image to "simmer" through the day so at night it serves as a bridge for desire and initiation.

SEXUAL FANTASIES

Sexual fantasies serve both as a bridge to desire and a means of enhancing eroticism. The wonderful thing about sexual fantasies is you can have them any way you like. You have the last word on casting, plot, direction, editing, camera angles, and special effects. Since you are the only person who sees your fantasies, you need not be afraid of censorship. As an accompaniment to masturbation sexual fantasies can be marvelously effective. A sexual fantasy can provide a pleasant interlude in

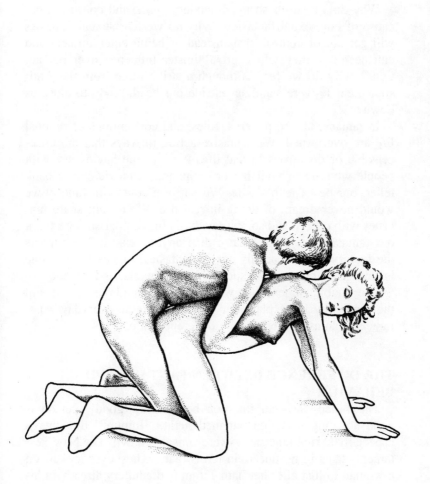

One of many positions for sexual intercourse. All too often only
one position is employed by a couple. Experimenting with positions facilitates sexual pleasure.

the middle of a tedious day. During intercourse, fantasy can transform a familiar sex partner into someone exotic, unattainable. Every sexual experience you ever wanted or wondered about can be yours through the magic of fantasy.

Why do we suffer so much anxiety, guilt, and confusion because of our sexual fantasies? Why do we fear sexual fantasies will get out of control, that instead of being entertainment and enhancement, they will exert a sinister influence over our actions? Why do we feel as though a strike force from the Anti-smut League were standing outside our head, ready to close us down?

In fantasy, all the patterns, rules, and conventions of rational life are overturned. We fantasize acting in ways that are unacceptable or disastrous in real life. We imagine having sex with people who are unavailable or peripheral: a movie star, a bank teller, our best friend's wife. We perform actions in fantasy we would never dream of doing in real life. We do not share fantasies with others, and so, with no basis for comparison, we think our fantasies are more bizarre than anyone else's. The truth is the fantasy life (especially sexual fantasies) of nearly everyone is strange, unpredictable, socially unacceptable, and chaotic.

The trouble comes when we try to understand our fantasies in the same way we explain our ordered, rational, everyday experiences. Fantasies are a totally different realm.

THE DIFFERENCE BETWEEN FANTASY AND BEHAVIOR

The Judeo-Christian tradition believes a "good" person is good not only in action but in thought. "Impure" thoughts—especially sexual fantasies—were considered evil. The New Testament states in no uncertain terms that "whosoever lookest on a woman to lust after her hath committed adultery already in his heart." This blurs the crucially important distinction between thought and action, between fantasy and reality. A psychologically healthy attitude allows us to be comfortable with our fantasy life and use fantasies to promote desire, arousal, and orgasm.

There is confusion about valid roles for sexual fantasy. We are unsure whether, or to what extent, fantasies represent what we actually want to do or are capable of doing. Do a married man's fantasies of having sex with another woman mean he does not find his wife sexually desirable? Do a man's fantasies of rape mean he is in danger of committing sexual assault? Do a heterosexual's fantasies of sex with men mean he is homosexual? These questions cause anxiety and confusion.

The core is the profound difference between fantasizing about doing something and actually doing it. Almost everyone has aggressive, antisocial, and bizarre sexual fantasies, but very few people act these out. The danger of antisocial fantasies is not the behavior but the guilt feelings they engender. Guilt is a powerful and self-defeating emotion. Sexual fantasies do not control a person's behavior, but guilt and obsessiveness as a result of these fantasies have a strong impact. Guilt serves as a negative force that keeps a person obsessively focused on a particular fantasy. It makes us uncomfortable with our sexual feelings. Guilt lowers a man's sexual self-esteem and discourages communication between partners.

In coming to terms with our sexual fantasies, we should not try to "purify" our thoughts or impose rigid control, but use fantasies to promote desire and eroticism. As for guilt, it has no positive use whatsoever.

MISUSE OF FANTASIES

When a particular thought or idea is associated with guilt, fear, or anxiety, it takes on a power and importance it should not have. It becomes obsessive and controlling. In some cases, an obsessive fantasy assumes central focus, displacing other forms of sexual desire. The fantasy produces intense arousal, but also intense guilt—a very unhealthy combination of emotions. For example, a man who has intense, guilt-laden fantasies about exposing himself to girls and becomes obsessed with that fantasy, is in big trouble. The combination of guilt and compulsion results in the man's developing a pedophiliac arousal pattern which functions in a compulsive, addictive manner. Another example is a fetish arousal pattern, the centering of sexual feelings on an inanimate object, which then becomes the sole stimulus capable of triggering sexual response. Fetishists are portrayed humorously as roguish gentlemen gloating lasciviously over their collections of women's shoes or lace panties. But fetishism is a sad affair in real life, it represents a severe limitation on the man's sexual life. His obsession with women's underwear is not problematic because it is morally wrong; it is problematic because it is the only thing he has, because it controls his sexual expression. Fetishism, exhibitionism, or pedophilia are extreme forms of fantasies that are compulsively acted out. These are the exceptions, not the rule. The intervention is to break the pattern of guilt-laden, obsessive sexual fantasies and compulsive sexual behavior.

The best strategy with regard to sexual fantasy is not to suppress your erotic imaginings or reject socially unacceptable fantasies, but to deliberately cultivate as widely varied a repertoire as you find enjoyable. To return to the cinematic metaphor, it makes little sense to watch the same film over and over again when you have at your disposal the enormous resources of a private Hollywood. Whatever erotic entertainments we fantasize, the vast majority of us are in no danger of behaviorally wandering outside the bounds of acceptable sexual behavior. There is no such thing as an unhealthy sexual fantasy, as long as it remains a fantasy and doesn't become obsessive or acted out in a compulsive, self-defeating manner.

POSITIVE FUNCTIONS OF FANTASY

Sexual fantasies are normal and healthy, serving several purposes. We need an occasional vacation from the rationality of everyday life, and fantasy provides just that. Dreams are a common mode of our fantasy lives—just about everyone dreams. In the course of an average night's sleep, two to three hours are spent dreaming. People deprived of dreaming become irritable and depressed.

When the content of our dreams contain themes of a bizarre or antisocial nature, we react by making the same mistake we do with waking fantasies—we blur the dividing line between fantasy and reality. Bizarre sexual dreams are very common—dreams of incest, of homosexuality, intercourse with a variety of sexually proscribed personages ranging from one's mother-in-law to the family dog. One dream that many men find disturbing—having intercourse with a hermaphrodite, a woman who has a penis—is a common motif found in the art and literature of many cultures. Don't expect dreams and fantasies to be rational or make sense. Accept your dreams and fantasies. It's normal to have abnormal sexual fantasies.

Sexual fantasies differ from dreams in that they occur during waking life, when we have conscious control and are able to choose fantasy themes. If we keep in mind the distinction between fantasy and reality, between thought and act, then fantasy can be a way of indulging in wishes and desires that are inappropriate or unacceptable in real life.

Two common fantasies when a man sees an attractive woman are to imagine what she would look like naked and what it would be like to have sex with her. Men experience a conflict between their professed attitudes of respect for women and the content of their fantasies, but if the distinction between enjoying a fantasy and actually engaging in a behavior is kept in mind, you can enjoy the fantasy without guilt or anxiety. Having such fantasies does not mean you are a male chauvinist who wants to rape every woman you see. A man can have an active fantasy life that contradicts every personal ethic he subscribes to without violating his values in terms of behavior. By their nature, sexual fantasies involve socially unacceptable sexual activity. Almost no one fantasizes about sex with his wife in his bedroom in the missionary position.

Fantasy can enhance a dating relationship. Sexual fantasies can be a source of excitement and strengthen desire. This is true whether the relationship is new or long-standing, whether intimate or at the flirtation stage. Married men could improve their sexual life by incorporating erotic activities with their wives into their fantasies. For example, fantasize about being sexual with her in a special, sexy outfit. Some couples enjoy sharing sexual fantasies. Telling your wife about a fantasy in which she comes to your office and seduces you can heighten erotic feelings— though it is highly unlikely you would want to act out this fantasy, unless you have a very private office.

Sexual fantasies can enhance a relationship in another, quite different way. Fantasy can serve as a rehearsal, which may be particularly helpful for younger males. He rehearses an entire lovemaking scene, revising and editing. As a result, the real-life event is more comfortable and he's more confident.

Fantasy is used as an accompaniment during intercourse. In

fact, 75 percent of men fantasize during partner sex. Fantasies serve as a bridge to greater arousal. Imagining sex with a different woman is a common fantasy, yet most men feel guilt about indulging in this fantasy. Such guilt is unnecessary, however, since changing a partner's identity in your imagination does not mean you want to change it in real life. One of Barry's students liked to evoke a fantasy of multiple sex partners during intercourse with his wife. He imagined six women, one of whom was his wife, were making love to him. Two would take turns sucking on his penis, another would move her finger in and out of his anus, a fourth would suck on his nipples, a fifth presents her vulva for him to explore with his tongue, and a sixth would wildly rub her body against his. Other images would flit in and out of his mind, such as two women making love or three women fighting to give him fellatio. Far from being guilt provoking, these fantasies served to heighten arousal during marital sex.

Bizarre and antisocial fantasy themes are normal. There is no need to feel guilty or disturbed about the content of any fantasy as long as it does not become obsessive or acted out. It is natural, for example, to fantasize about having sex with women of a different race or ethnic group. Group sex, anal sex, forced sex, observing others having sex, and sadomasochistic experiences are common fantasy themes. Violent and aggressive sexual fantasies are quite common. Homosexual fantasies are normal, too. Homosexual fantasies are the fourth most common theme among heterosexual men and heterosexual fantasies are the third most common theme among homosexual men. Tom, a student of Barry's, occasionally utilized a homosexual fantasy. While masturbating, he would imagine there were two handsome, muscular men who were his sexual slaves. One would perform anal intercourse while the other gave him oral sex. Although he found the fantasy quite arousing, it was not something he wanted to carry through to behavior. He accepted homosexuality as valid for gay people, but he was a satisfied heterosexual.

Sexual fantasies, rather than being something to fear and avoid, can be a source of great pleasure. No fantasy is ''sick'' or ''immoral'' as long as it remains a fantasy. The danger is not the fantasy itself but the guilt that accompanies it. It is guilt that makes us focus obsessively on one fantasy. Barry's clinical experience has shown the healthiest and most rewarding practice is to cultivate a number of different fantasies, enjoy them all, and feel guilty about none of them. Fantasy can serve to amuse, excite, educate, and refresh us. Fantasies serve as a bridge to increase involvement and arousal during partner sex. Fantasy makes the experience of being a sexual male richer and more satisfying.

ORAL SEX

Consider the mouth. What a marvelously sensitive and expressive part of the body it is. Our mouths have a wonderful ability to receive sensations. Best of all, our mouths have an enormous capacity for experiencing pleasure. Think of the enjoyment of biting into a juicy apple or downing a chilled beer on a sweltering day.

Like our mouths, our genitals are richly supplied with nerve endings and exquisitely receptive to pleasurable sensations. Isn't it natural and fitting that, in seeking to experience and impart sexual pleasure, we employ oral-genital stimulation? Our mouths and our genitals, which have so much in common and so much to offer one another, can unite to produce a very special and intense pleasure.

We are accustomed to using our mouths, lips, and tongues, to kiss, suck, lick, nibble, and bite the lips, face, breasts, and other parts of our partner's body. Oral-genital stimulation is a normal extension of oral stimulation. It is a coming together of the two most sensitive pleasure-giving and pleasure-receiving areas of the body. This is equally true of fellatio (oral stimulation of the penis) and cunnilingus (oral stimulation of the vulva). Both are natural and healthy activities. Couples who enjoy oral sex rate their sexual lives more satisfying than couples who avoid oral sex because of discomfort, inhibition, or believing the myth that it's a perverse behavior.

MYTHS ABOUT ORAL SEX

Unfortunately, a whole complex of prejudices and misconceptions have grown up around the subject of oral sex, causing people to feel conflicted about it and anxious or guilty when they do it. Let us confront these negative attitudes and dispel the myths and inhibitions that prevent oral sex from being freely and comfortably experienced.

A major misconception is that oral sex is unclean. Americans in particular have a concern, practically an obsession, with oral cleanliness, reflected in the endless succession of ads for toothpaste, mouthwashes, and breath mints. The genitals are considered a "dirty" part of the body, not only because of puritanical attitudes but because of the close connection between the sex organs and the organs of excretion. The male urethra serves as a channel for both semen and urine. The female expels urine through the urethral meatus, located between the clitoris and vagina. Many people are concerned by the prospect of taking into the mouth organs that have been contaminated by urine.

Such concerns are unfounded. Many people prefer to wash their genitals before engaging in sexual activity, especially oral sex. With ordinary hygiene, the genitals are as germ free and clean smelling as any part of the body. In fact, the mouth contains more germs than the penis or vulva. Sexual secretions—the male's semen and female lubrication—are antiseptic and harmless protein substances. Negative attitudes are caused by ignorance of the structure and function of the genitals—your own and those of your partner. Self-examination and mutual exploration of the genital area can be an enlightening and liberating experience.

One of Barry's clients, a young, married law student who had been very active sexually and proud of his sexual prowess, experienced such a breakthrough. He very much enjoyed being fellated, but was uncomfortable with cunnilingus and would avoid doing it even if his wife requested it. Not surprisingly, this created sexual imbalance and tension in their relationship. Originally, they had come for therapy to reduce anxiety about childbirth. As therapy progressed, the strife caused by his attitude toward oral sex emerged as a significant problem. He felt disgusted by the fact the urethra was located in the vulva area. "Piss doesn't turn me on," was the way he expressed it. At Barry's suggestion, he agreed to make a thorough visual inspection of his wife's genitals. This exercise was a turning point. He realized that while the urethra was indeed located in the vulva area, he could avoid it by concentrating on the clitoral shaft and inner lips. His anxiety was reduced considerably, and he was able to enjoy giving oral stimulation. He found it particularly arousing if she fellated him at the same time.

This example shows not only the value of knowledge in overcoming hang-ups, but the importance of choice in oral sex (or any form of sexuality). While therapy techniques can be helpful in changing attitudes and behavior, don't allow yourself to be forced by outside pressure (including this book) into sexual activity you feel uncomfortable with. Our sex lives should be motivated by a genuine desire to experiment and increase sources of pleasure, not by a sense of duty or to prove you are sexually liberated. You may decide oral sex is not for you, but why not be adventurous and give it a fair chance?

Vaginal secretions have a definite flavor of their own—a salty, tangy, complex taste that is not quite like anything else. Many men enjoy this taste and find it highly arousing. Others may not find it quite so appealing. While it is useless to try to persuade someone to like something he does not, it is true tastes may be acquired, particularly when the surrounding circumstances are positive.

The key to learning to enjoy cunnilingus is to approach it in a comfortable, gradual manner. For example, he might begin by kissing her vulva with his lips closed. When he feels comfortable, he can progress to using his tongue and open mouth. There are several products on the market—flavored vaginal sprays—that appeal to men who have ambivalent feelings about oral sex. Some of these products are of dubious value from a health point of view, increasing the risk for vaginal infections. Only use those which are hypoallergenic. Other men feel it would be more honest to cultivate an appreciation for the real thing rather than try to make it palatable with synthetic peppermint.

Oral sex has been unjustly maligned in many ways. A common misconception is that men who enjoy fellatio are trying to avoid intercourse. A frequent contention is oral sex is a sign of immaturity—based on the idea that heterosexual intercourse in the male-on-top position is the only truly ''adult'' form of sexuality. This is nonsense. The hallmark of healthy sexuality is the ability to experiment and communicate to enhance pleasure and eroticism. Couples who limit their sexual activity to a single method or position are not proving their maturity; they are stuck in a rut. Lack of imagination increases the possibility of becoming bored with sex and developing inhibited sexual desire. Oral sex adds variety and eroticism to the couple's sex life. Surveys show couples who engage in oral sex report greater sexual satisfaction. Approximately 85 percent of couples experiment with oral sex and 40 percent use it regularly. Men who report the highest satisfaction enjoy both receiving fellatio and giving cunnilingus.

THE RELATIONSHIP BETWEEN ORAL SEX AND INTERCOURSE

Some men believe the use of the mouth in sex is indicative of a lack of virility. The assumption—based on a narrow and rigid concept of sex—is that a man who orally stimulates a woman does so because he is incapable of satisfying her with his penis. Actually, a man who incorporates cunnilingus into his sexual repertoire is likely to be more comfortable and secure sexually. He is more confident, both in intercourse and oral sex, than a man who limits his lovemaking.

A surprising number of men fear a woman might become "addicted" to oral sex. It is true many women find oral sex extremely pleasurable since it provides direct stimulation of the clitoral area, but they do not become indifferent to intercourse. On the contrary, couples who use oral sex are more likely to enjoy other sexual techniques, including most definitely, intercourse. Intercourse and oral sex are complementary, not either-or, activities. Couples use fellatio and cunnilingus as pleasuring activities that lead to, and indeed whet the appetite for, intercourse.

Seeing oral sex as a natural, healthy, and enhancing activity is essential to deriving optimal pleasure from it. Too often, men think of oral sex as a forbidden pleasure they must procure either by coercion or outside the marriage. The prevalence of this is demonstrated by married men going to prostitutes for fellatio, not intercourse. These men set up a strict dichotomy between the kind of sex allowed within marriage (only intercourse) and the sex they seek outside of marriage (where anything goes). There is no reason why such a dichotomy should exist. The

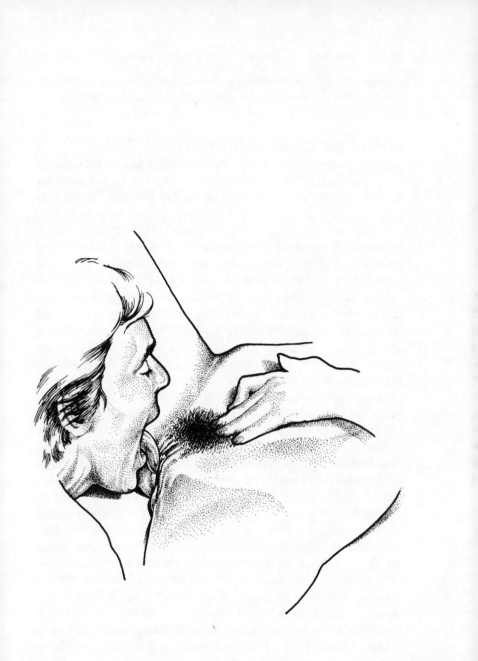

Cunnilingus. We often forget just how marvelously sensitive and expressive the mouth is.

mistaken belief that there are sexual activities which are not permissible for married couples perpetuates sexual dissatisfaction.

COMMUNICATING ABOUT ORAL SEX

Many couples try oral sex, but give up when it does not go well. The man tells himself since she does not seem turned on, he is doing her a favor by not asking her to continue. Such an attitude denies the woman's potential responsiveness as well as ignoring the complexity of fellatio and cunnilingus as sexual behaviors that require communication, comfort, guidance, and feedback. If couples reacted to their first intercourse as they do to their first attempts at oral sex, they would give up intercourse.

Oral sex is something a man has a perfect right to request, just as she has a perfect right to request it from him. They both should feel comfortable asking for oral stimulation, and guiding one another in developing satisfying oral sex scenarios and techniques. A genuine give and take (using both verbal and nonverbal communication) will enable the couple to find ways of pleasing each other. Men think of fellatio as a "symbolic" act rather than a mutually pleasurable activity. They feel just getting their partner to "go down on them" is all they can expect.

The point is well illustrated by a couple in sex therapy. The man had pressed his wife to fellate him, but she could not get up the courage. Finally, he got her to do it one evening when she was drunk. After overcoming the initial resistance, she repeated the act on a regular basis. However, he offered no feedback or guidance. She worked out a method of fellating him, according to what seemed arousing to her. Rather than taking the glans of the penis into her mouth, she concentrated on sucking and stimulating the shaft. When Barry asked the man whether he was satisfied he became embarrassed. "Don't tell my wife," he said, "but I dislike her technique—it hurts!" He agreed to communicate this and request experimenting with other techniques. Eventually they worked out a style of oral stimulation that was mutually satisfying.

Problems with oral sex arise because of a failure to communicate. For example, many women fear gagging on the penis. Rather than demanding she continue despite her discomfort or withdrawing out of a misplaced sense of compassion, the appropriate response is to encourage her to experiment until she is able to comfortably engage in fellatio. She could place the penis to one side of her mouth rather than in the center or hold the shaft in her fingers as she takes it into her mouth. These techniques give her greater control and prevent the penis from going so deep that the gag reflex is triggered. A nondemand atmosphere is best for developing comfort and skill. The ability to laugh can be invaluable for relieving awkwardness. After all, sex—of whatever variety—is supposed to be fun!

Another issue is the woman's discomfort over the man's ejaculating in her mouth or her reluctance to swallow semen once he ejaculates. Some men feel that by rejecting his semen she is rejecting him. Here, again, we encounter a rigid approach to oral sex and a failure to honestly and empathically communicate feelings. The woman allowing him to ejaculate in her mouth or swallowing his semen is not the chief factor in his pleasure. Our focus in sex should be pleasure, not symbolism or performance. The woman's willingness or unwillingness relates to what is comfortable and pleasurable for her, not to acceptance or rejection of him. There is no reason to expect fellatio to follow a set format. Whether fellatio is used as a pleasuring technique or continues to orgasm can be decided according to what is pleasurable for both partners.

Awareness and communication are just as important for cunnilingus. Men who are not aware of their partner's sexual sensitivities or have not received guidance from her may do oral stimulation in ways that are ineffective. The man might focus his attention on the vagina or outer lips, where the concentration of nerve endings is sparse. Or he might stimulate the clitoris in a way that is too direct or rough, causing more pain than pleasure.

The clitoris is an extremely sensitive organ, particularly at the tip (glans). Most women prefer indirect stimulation around the clitoral shaft rather than a direct focus on the glans. Women respond to different types of oral stimulation. Some like slow, rhythmic stroking, others prefer a rapid, focused movement. Still others like the man to run his tongue over the clitoris and then suck on the clitoral shaft and labia. Women can be extremely responsive to oral stimulation, but only when they are already aroused. Cunnilingus when the woman is minimally aroused is usually counterproductive. Discuss the kind of stimulation she prefers and follow her guidance. Each partner has the right—in fact, the responsibility—to request stimulation that is pleasurable and erotic. Sexual requests are best when they are clear and direct, without pressure or threats of negative consequences inherent in demands.

ENJOYING ORAL SEX

To improve comfort and pleasure with oral sex, begin with manual genital stimulation. One partner takes the role of giver and the other recipient. Begin oral stimulation gradually, concentrating at first on the insides of the thighs and the area surrounding the genitals. Gradually move to oral-genital stimulation, experimenting with different types of movements such as licking, sucking, kissing, and a darting tongue movement. Keep the lines of communication open regarding comfort and pleasure; each partner is free to say what he likes and doesn't like. Once you feel comfortable with oral sex, there is no end to possible variations. Many couples find mutual, simultaneous oral stimulation—the ''69'' position—to be extremely satisfying. Others find they are not comfortable receiving and giving stimulation at the same time, they prefer taking turns. Some people like oral sex best in the position where one is standing and the other is kneeling, others enjoy it best when one is lying down and the other kneels above. Some enjoy being passive while receiving oral sex, with the giver doing the movement, others find it more arousing to move when being stimulated. The key to effective, satisfying oral sex is comfort and communication.

The reason for engaging in oral sex is to enhance pleasure, not prove something to yourself or the partner. Be wary of the new sexual conformism in which people feel pressure to show they are free of inhibitions by demonstrating readiness to engage in every possible form of sexual behavior. A particular sexual technique becomes the ''in'' thing, and people who think of themselves as sexually liberated feel they must do it. The latest of these sexual fashions are anilingus, the oral stimulation of the anus, and oral stimulation of the testicles, taking the whole testicle into the mouth. There is nothing abnormal or ''bad'' about these techniques as long as proper hygiene is utilized and care

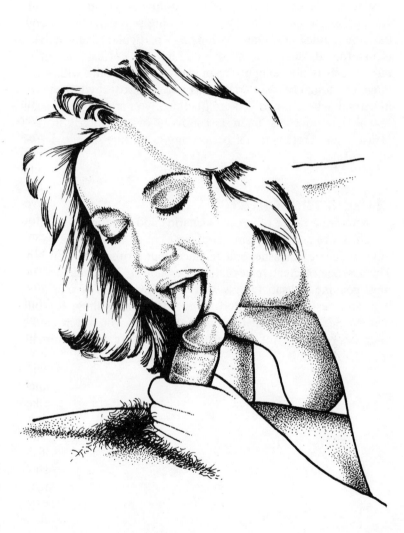

Fellatio. The enjoyment of receiving oral stimulation.

is taken not to hurt the partner. What is unhealthy is to engage in these techniques because it is expected or you fear being labeled inhibited or unsophisticated.

Whether the sexual experience is anilingus, group sex, bondage and discipline, swinging, or watching pornographic videos, the same guideline applies. As long as a particular sexual activity is not forced, does not involve children, is not carried out in public, and is not compulsive or destructive, it falls within the range of normal sexual variation. If you feel pressured to engage in certain acts to prove you are liberated, you are not expressing sexuality in your best interest. The focus of sexuality is sharing pleasure and eroticism, not performing according to an external standard.

CLOSING THOUGHTS

There are a range of sexual scenarios and techniques that can enrich desire and eroticism. You can explore and choose variations which add pleasure and enhance your intimate relationship. The essence of creative sexuality does not lie in technique. The most genuine and satisfying sex involves awareness of your feelings and desires and comfort in communicating these to your partner. Sex is most creative and erotic when you are aware of your desires, those of your partner, and share as an intimate couple.

11

BEING A CARING MALE AND
A NURTURING PARENT

Males are cast in the role of uncaring and uninvolved bystanders in the conception, birth, and parenting process. Traditionally, this is the domain of women. Fathers are represented as bumblers whose only contribution is the sperm that starts things off. This myth has been portrayed in countless novels, movies, and TV shows. The standard scene shows the wife's announcement she is pregnant and the husband's astonished response. The decision to have a baby, her missed period, and pregnancy test have all gone on without his knowledge. When labor begins he paces the waiting room pestering the nurse with idiotic questions. Presented with the baby, he is afraid to hold him. If it is a boy, he brings a football or baseball to the hospital. If it is a girl, he does nothing, for it is assumed he has nothing to teach her. His only task will be to provide for her and protect her from predatory males.

Throughout the process the male is portrayed as not only peripheral but superfluous. The theme is clear: women and women alone are responsible for all decisions about conception, childbirth and rearing of children.

No man should allow his role as an involved, caring spouse and nurturing father to be negated. Fatherhood is one of life's unparalleled experiences, providing emotional rewards of a unique caliber. Because the experience is potentially such a rich and fulfilling one, it should be undergone deliberately, consciously, purposefully. Only by participating fully can he take advantage of the opportunities for emotional satisfaction that being a caring man and parent offers. A man should choose fatherhood, savoring all that it has to offer, rather than passively acquiescing.

CHOOSING NOT TO HAVE A CHILD

But choosing fatherhood means a man must have the option of choosing not to be a father. Before the widespread use of contraception, before the population explosion, before the opening of the job market to women, it was taken for granted that soon after a couple married they would have children. Today, there is no reason to make this assumption. Having children is a choice, not an obligation. It is not valid or realistic to insist the purpose of sex is procreation. Sex is the way we conceive children, but this is an optional function, not a required one. The major functions of marital sex are to share pleasure, reinforce intimacy, and be a tension reducer to deal with the hassles of life and marriage. Sex for pleasure and intimacy is normal, healthy, and worthwhile. Couples should not feel guilty about enjoying sex for its own sake. They do not have to produce babies in order to justify their marriage, their sexuality, or to please their parents and make them grandparents.

There are good reasons to decide not to have children. A child is a major financial investment. Hospital bills, visits to the doctor, baby clothes and furniture entail sizable expenditures. As the child grows the expenses become even larger. Clothing, schooling, toys, entertainment, medical and dental costs, and college tuition add up to an ever-increasing amount. The addition of a child will reduce the amount of money the couple have and lower their standard of living.

Some couples are hesitant to have a baby because it means the wife would give up or scale back her career (either temporarily or permanently). Of course, an alternative would be for the wife to continue her career while the husband stayed home. In some cases this might work, although it's quite rare. The norm for two career families is to hire professional help to care for the child or use a child care center. But even with such assistance, the strain of raising a child while balancing two careers is considerable, especially for couples in their twenties. The pressure causes something to give, either the marriage or the woman's career.

Couples who relish their freedom and companionship might be unwilling to upset this balance by introducing a third member. Babies cut down enormously on time and energy available. Couples who consider their social life and fun times indispensable should think seriously about the consequences before having a child.

Some couples decide not to have children simply because they don't particularly like children. Not being fond of children isn't something to be ashamed of. It doesn't imply a person lacks warmth. If you don't like or feel comfortable with children, it makes little sense to become a parent.

Having a child represents a long-term commitment—for at least eighteen years parents are responsible for the child's welfare. A couple should take a long, sober look at this commitment and consider realistically all the obligations and limitations involved before becoming pregnant. There are positive aspects of remaining childless, including freedom to travel, try alternative lifestyles, and live where they please rather than choosing a neighborhood because of schools and child-related activities. There is an increasing acceptance of couples weighing the advantages and disadvantages of childbearing and choosing childlessness.

CHOOSING FATHERHOOD

If a man chooses to have a child after thoroughly discussing this with his wife, his involvement has only begun. The major reason to choose fatherhood is it is one of life's special experiences. If the decision were based solely on practical or financial factors, the rational choice would be to remain childless. The couple make an emotional commitment to the process of having and raising a child.

The next decision is when to have a child. Ideally the birth of a child is the result of planning rather than accident or chance. The transition from being a couple to being a family is no small event. It places demands on the man and woman which dramatically change their lives. It is preferable the child be wanted, planned, and expected.

One of the most important guidelines is to wait at least two years after marriage before having a child. This allows you to strengthen and reinforce your marital bond. The decision to become a family acknowledges this is a viable, stable marriage. When the couple choose to have a child and are aware of the work and stress as well as joy and satisfaction, they are better prepared to parent. Unfortunately, family planning is not as widely practiced as people believe. Four of ten children born to married couples are not planned, and one in four brides is pregnant at the time of marriage (or already has a child). For teenage brides, the proportion is much greater.[8]

FERTILITY PROBLEMS

About 20 percent of couples have difficulty conceiving. Of these, 70 percent will eventually conceive if they receive competent medical help. The couple with a fertility problem need not feel embarrassed or abnormal. Consult a fertility specialist (gynecologist, endocrinologist or urologist) to determine possible causes in *both* the man and the woman. Fertility interventions have become more sophisticated and effective. Be an active and aware patient and work cooperatively with the specialist.

It is crucial to be clear about the difference between infertility and sexuality. Infertility means the couple (the problem may be traced to the man, the woman, or both) is having difficulty conceiving. This has nothing to do with the man's sexual prowess, his identity as a male, or his ability to function as a lover. Fertility problems are stressful enough without adding inappropriate feelings of sexual deficit or failure. A man or woman who is biologically unable to have a child is still a fully functioning sexual person.

Infertility is one of the most stressful problems a couple encounters. The process of an infertility workup (taking basal temperature, having intercourse on a rigid schedule, going for continual tests and appointments, surgical procedures) is time consuming, expensive and psychologically draining. Their life is organized around the fertility problem. Each month is an emotional roller coaster of high hopes and bitter disappointment when the menstrual period arrives. When the problem involves the man's low sperm count or poor sperm motility (the sperm are slow swimmers), this threatens his self-esteem. Rationally, he knows it is a medical problem, not a measure of worth or masculinity, but emotionally he feels deficient. In 40 percent of fertility problems, male factors are a component. The varicocele operation is a standard intervention where the vein in the testicle is altered surgically to improve sperm motility. Medications and hormone pills are other possible medical interventions for males.

Couples who are unable to conceive have to carefully consider the alternatives: (1) remain childless; (2) adopt; (3) utilize artificial insemination with husband or donor sperm; and (4) *in vitro* fertilization. In making this decision, thoughtful discussion between themselves, with the physician, family and close friends, and a professional counselor is advised.

TIMING OF CHILDREN

When should a couple have children? There isn't a hard-and-fast rule, but waiting at least two years after marriage is strongly advised. It takes at least this long for the couple to develop an intimate, secure bond. This gives them time to create a couple style based on understanding each other's feelings, habits, and preferences. When the baby comes, they are better able to work through the demands a child makes on their lives. A couple who conceive a child either before or slightly after the date of their marriage have the task of learning about and adjusting to a third and extremely demanding person when they have hardly begun to adjust to each other.

UNPLANNED PREGNANCIES

When we speak of family planning we do so with some qualification. Nothing in life goes 100 percent according to plan, including conception of a child. Accidents do happen, even to people who use contraception conscientiously. When a woman becomes pregnant accidentally, a decision must be made. Should they carry through with the unplanned pregnancy, keep the child or give it up for adoption, or have an abortion? Husband and wife need to face this choice together. An argument could be made that since the woman carries the child she should be the one to decide. It is the woman who must undergo childbirth or abortion, and this makes her feelings stronger and more immediate, but it is the man and woman together who will parent the child. The equity model of male-female relationships includes contraception, conception, abortion, and parenting.

Coming to a joint decision helps make the marriage closer. If the choice is abortion or giving the child up for adoption, sharing lessens the burden of regret. Abortion involves minor surgery for the woman and difficult psychological and emotional reactions for both people. It is not to be chosen lightly. The majority of couples decide, once having conceived, they now want the child. But if the addition of a child (a first or additional one) would have a negative effect on the marriage and family, for whatever reason—financial, physical, relational, or psychological—abortion or adoption may be the best alternatives. "There's always room for one more" is not a good guide to follow, sometimes there isn't. Being married does not obligate the couple to continue the pregnancy or keep the child. Approximately three of ten abortions are performed on married women. Couples choosing abortion can in the future conceive a planned, wanted child. If they decide they definitely don't want more children, they should seriously consider sterilization.

INVOLVEMENT WITH THE PREGNANCY

Once your wife becomes pregnant, several issues arise. Should you be involved in the pregnancy or be the sort of man portrayed in sitcoms? When was the last time you enjoyed something you weren't involved in? Being a bystander isn't much fun, so why not involve yourself wholeheartedly in the birth of your child?

Pregnancy cannot be physically shared. It can, however, be shared in other ways. The couple can jointly learn about pregnancy and visit the obstetrician together. They can take a prepared (also called natural childbirth or the Lamaze method) childbirth course. The woman learns and practices exercises to reduce and control pain. She is able to go through the birth process awake and conscious, without anesthesia. The husband functions as a "coach," helping her throughout labor and delivery. This allows him to become a functioning member of the delivery team and, more important, an active supporter for his wife.

Prepared childbirth can add immeasurably to the emotional satisfaction of the birth experience. For the woman it means the chance to experience the extraordinary process of childbirth while fully conscious with the support of a loving and trusted spouse who anticipates and responds to her needs. For the man, childbirth helps develop a deep attachment to his child and family. Barry being present for the birth of our children represented peak experiences in our lives.

CHANGES DURING PREGNANCY

No matter how deeply involved a man is in his wife's pregnancy, there is the most basic aspect of the process that cannot be shared—carrying and giving birth to the child. Pregnancy involves physical, hormonal, and emotional changes. While pregnant, a woman feels different from any way she has ever felt before. The man will never have the same experience. He may feel left out and have the childish, but very normal, feeling that she is not paying enough attention to his needs. This causes him to withdraw emotionally and sexually, creating a rift in their relationship.

Just as you find it hard to understand what she is going through, she may find it equally hard to understand your feelings. The answer is to communicate fears and hopes. It is your responsibility to share concerns or negative feelings, however silly or unmanly you think they are. Sharing negative as well as positive feelings makes the pregnancy experience more meaningful for both of you.

SEX DURING PREGNANCY

Pregnancy often interferes with the couple's sexual relationship. Fears about sex during pregnancy are unnecessary. Contrary to popular belief, a growing fetus is one of the most effectively protected objects in nature. It is fine to have intercourse throughout the pregnancy, including the last trimester, unless she experiences uterine bleeding, severe cramps or pain. Except for those rare cases where the obstetrician imposes restrictions (for example, where the woman has a history of miscarriage), pregnant couples can have an active sex life. In fact, during the second trimester, increased pelvic vasocongestion might facilitate sexual response.

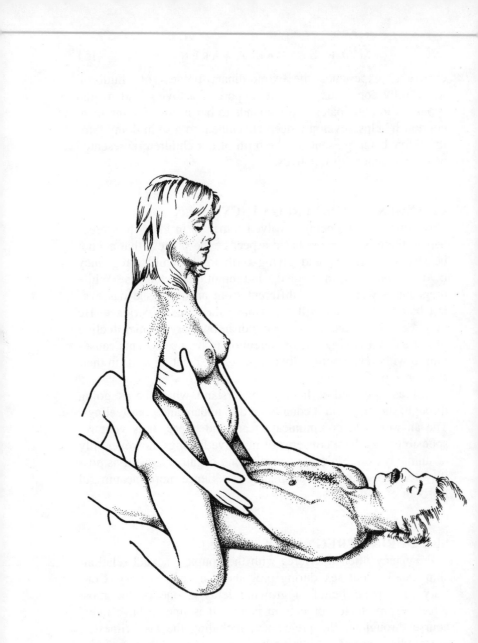

Intercourse during pregnancy. Except in rare cases, it is a myth that the fetus can be damaged by intercourse during pregnancy.

You are advised to change intercourse positions as the pregnancy enters the third trimester. As the woman's belly gets larger, the male on top position becomes increasingly uncomfortable. An excellent alternative is side rear entry intercourse. One of the best positions is the sitting-kneeling position in which the woman sits (pillows supporting her lower back) with her buttocks resting at the edge of the couch (chair or bed) and her feet on the floor. The man kneels between her legs. He puts pillows under his knees in order to bring his genitals to the same height as the woman's vulva so he can enter comfortably. This is an excellent position since it not only alleviates pressure on her stomach, but allows the partners to touch, caress, and communicate during intercourse. Many couples prefer a slower, more gentle style of intercourse which these positions lend themselves to. Each couple should experiment to find the position and style of being sexual they are comfortable with.

Childbirth is a strenuous process, causing severe soreness in the vaginal area. When an episiotomy (an incision to widen the vaginal opening) is performed, this takes time to heal. Physicians advise couples to refrain from intercourse for four to six weeks after childbirth because of pain and risk of infection. This ban on intercourse in addition to sleep deprivation and the stresses of caring for a newborn may cause a husband and wife to become emotionally distant. In fact, a first pregnancy (the three months before or the three months after childbirth) is the most common time for a husband to begin an extramarital affair.

It is the period immediately following birth—when intercourse is impossible and the woman is very tired and devoting most of her available energy to mothering—that is the most trying. Rather than looking for sex outside the marriage, a healthier course of action is to speak to the spouse about your feelings. This is a time for both husband and wife to lean on and derive support from their relationship, not allow it to fade away. The husband who cares about preserving the quality of his marriage will alter his sex life so it will not endanger the marital bond. He could use masturbation to achieve the sexual release he desires or ask her to manually stimulate or fellate him. He worries she has enough to concern her and does not want to be bothered by his sexual needs, but in most cases this is not true. Expressing his desire reassures her she is important and he continues to find her attractive.

Wendy and Phil

Wendy and Phil had been in therapy for a sexual dysfunction, which they overcame. They found out how important it was to maintain sensual and sexual connection when Wendy became pregnant. Phil, an enlisted man in the Army, was an unassertive fellow who found it difficult to make requests of Wendy, especially involving sexuality. After their child was born and they'd stopped intercourse, Phil found it hard to ask Wendy to stimulate him to orgasm. Finally he did, but his lack of self-assurance made him unpersuasive. "What's the difference between me doing it and you doing it?" was Wendy's reaction. Phil explained when she manually stimulated him he could look at her, touch her, feel close to her. Phil's statement made Wendy aware how much he wanted to be with her. She felt she was "giving" to Phil and could enjoy his pleasure rather than being asked to mechanically "do him" by giving him a "hand job." There was an increase in affection, hugging, kissing, and caressing. The stressful months after the baby's arrival were easier because they felt like an intimate and parental team.

FATHERING THE BABY

Once he has gotten through the joys and difficulties of pregnancy and childbirth, there is no reason a man can't continue to participate fully by learning to care for the baby. Why be an occasional helper when you can be a fully involved partner in child care? This is contrary to the traditional image of the American father. But in this case, as in so many others, it is the traditional images that cheat us of the pleasures and emotional satisfactions available in life. It is perfectly natural to feel warmth and affection toward a baby, particularly when it is your own. Babies are adorable, they are incredibly soft, smell good (except when they need changing), and do amusing and endearing things. It is a human response, not just a female one, to want to hold, cuddle, talk to and play with a child. There is no reason why we should deny ourselves this pleasure because of the traditional notion that a "real man" does not show warmth and caring. A man can be nurturing and maintain his sense of masculinity. Nurturing and masculinity are complementary.

Caring for a child involves time and effort, but the rewards gained through closeness and feeling good about yourself as a father more than make up for the work involved. Tell your wife you want to participate in child care. She can help you learn what you need to know about diapering, feeding and bathing. If neither of you is knowledgeable, you could read on the subject, ask a friend or relative for help, or take a hands-on course in child care. This helps create a truly cohesive family. A further benefit is when the husband shoulders his share of the burden the wife has more energy and attention to devote to their emotional and sexual relationship.

POSITIVE ADJUSTMENT TO A CHILD

The birth of a child is one of the most exciting, yet stressful, periods in marriage. The work involved, along with the extra financial and emotional demands, places a considerable strain on the man and their marriage. In many cases a coolness, a sense of alienation, creeps into the relationship. Typically, couple time and sexual frequency decrease.

But none of this is necessary. The best way to prepare for a child is to go through all the steps together—from decisions about family planning to taking turns at diapering and administering 2:00 A.M. feedings. Caring for a child is too much for one person. In the past the woman received extensive help from her mother and other female relatives. But since extended families rarely are so available, this is not possible. This change can be our gain. As men we have a chance to participate in the wonder, excitement, and emotional thrill of birth and being an involved, nurturing parent. Guiding and sharing in the growth and development of another human being can be one of the most emotionally rewarding experiences of your life. It's not an opportunity to let slip away.

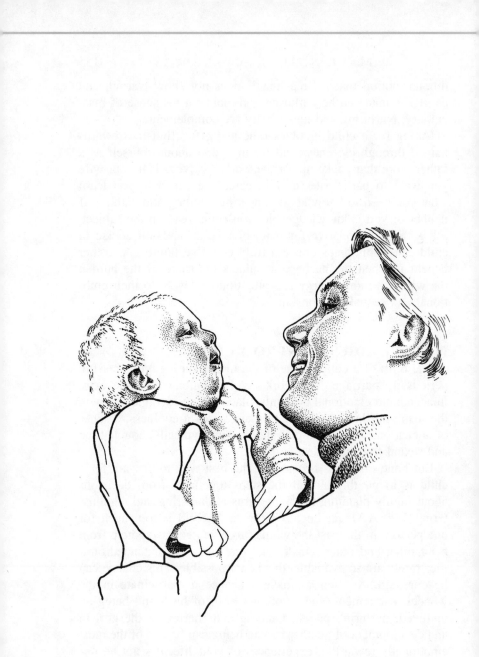

An expression of paternal affection. Unfortunately fathers tend not to continue physical contact as the child becomes older.

BEING A SEX EDUCATOR FOR YOUR CHILD

Obstetricians remark a newborn baby will have his first erection before the doctor has time to tie off the umbilical cord. Sex is a natural physiological process from the day we are born to the day we die. Research demonstrates babies have erections *in utero*. It doesn't take long for babies to discover sexuality. Babies, both male and female, quickly find they can produce pleasurable sensations by touching their genitals.

During the child's early development, sexual sensations are not distinguished from other pleasurable feelings. Children become aroused by experiences that are not specifically sexual (and so do adults—more often than we admit). An individual's sexual identity, feelings about his body, feelings about his genitals—components of his personality destined to play such an important role in later life—are in the process of formation. Children are not asexual, they are learning to be sexual. Sexuality itself—the raw material—is there from the start.

PARENTS AS MODELS

Children learn about sexuality partly through modeling. The earliest and most formative models are his parents. Our sexual patterns, hang-ups, feelings about our bodies, personal and sexual identities are connected with family learning experiences. This puts a great deal of responsibility on a parent. Parents want the best for their children, which includes a desire for them to have a healthy sexual self-esteem. But we cannot help children gain this unless we ourselves develop a positive attitude toward sexuality.

Most men feel their sex education was poor or nonexistent, focusing on the negative. Be aware of uncomfortable areas and help your child deal with his development better than you did as a child. The effort we put into developing our sexual awareness and improving marital sexuality pays off in two ways. First, we reap the benefits in terms of pleasure and emotional satisfaction. Second, we become good role models for our children, helping set them on the road toward an aware and self-accepting sexuality.

Few of us had sex educations that were nurturing or positive. The majority of today's adults grew up in homes where nudity was prohibited, masturbation brought severe reprimands, and discussion about sex was confined to a brief, uncomfortable five- or ten-minute talk between father and son. No real information was conveyed, just a vague admonition to "stay out of trouble." School sex education was absent or rudimentary, and the only religious sex education involved guilt and hearing "no." Whatever information you received came from peers, television, sex magazines, pornographic movies, or what you puzzled out for yourself.

FATHER-CHILD RELATIONSHIP

As men, we have an added difficulty in achieving a healthy self-esteem—one that stems from the lack of warmth and communication between boys and their fathers. Research indicates both boys and girls report being closer to their mothers than their fathers. Women report feeling closer to their children and enjoying parenting more than men. Boys and their fathers interact only within certain defined contexts such as sports or camping trips. A boy needs a sense of what it is to be a man. It is difficult to develop this unless he can talk with his father about feelings, ask questions about changes in his body, masturbation, the meaning of erections, conception and contraception, sexually transmitted diseases, and attitudes toward women.

A clear identity as a male (which needs to be established by age three) facilitates the boy's experimenting with "nonmasculine" activities such as playing house, taking care of babies, and cooking. The father feeling comfortable engaging in child-care activities as well as cooking and cleaning provides an excellent, realistic male model. As long as the boy has a solid male identity, he can enjoy individual choice and flexibility regarding activities and interests. He feels equally masculine playing the violin as playing sports. A secure and solid sense of maleness is the foundation upon which a boy can accept his growing sexual awareness.

Girls, too, need a close relationship with their father in order to grow into a full and healthy sense of themselves as females. One of the saddest things in our culture is the separation between father and daughter that widens as she enters adolescence. She needs as much as ever to feel love, support, affection, and recognition of herself as a person from both father and mother. However, father avoids her because he feels uncomfortable dealing with his daughter as a young woman and her developing sexuality.

PARENTS AS SEX EDUCATORS

As fathers we have the responsibility of guiding the awakening sexuality of our children. It is especially challenging because we live in a time of changing and confusing sexual mores. The puritanical equation of sex with sin and the double standard are weakening. This leaves parents in an ambiguous position and makes it hard for them to provide positive, realistic guidelines for their children.

Parents may be too liberal in one situation and too restrictive in another. Since it is a parent's job to set limits of acceptable and unacceptable behavior, being aware of the impact on a child's psychological and sexual development is particularly important. The guidelines we suggest are based on research data, clinical experience, or developed through parenting our children and grandchild. Sexual attitudes and values differ from family to family. It is possible to be overly lax in setting guidelines about sexuality, just as it is to be overly restrictive. Between these extremes are a range of healthy and constructive parental attitudes and child-rearing practices. It's important to raise a child to be comfortable with his sexuality.

FATHERS AND AFFECTION

Men feel more inhibition about showing affection with their children than do women. Fathers allow themselves to express affection with infants and young children, but beyond this stage, a father's hugs, kisses, and words of love become few and far between. Father's display of affection diminishes in direct proportion to his children's growing consciousness of him as a person. A child (as well as an adolescent and young adult) never outgrows the need to feel his parents love and care for him. If a parent ceases to express his love physically or verbally, the child has no way of knowing the love still exists.

Many children are aware their fathers love them only because mothers tell them ("You know your father loves you very much"), usually to counteract evidence to the contrary such as a spanking or being yelled at. The father's coldness is justified as an aspect of the traditional male role: it is the woman's place to be affectionate with the children, not the man's. His role is disciplinarian and task enforcer, to ensure they grow up to be competent, successful human beings. This lack of affection between a man and his children cheats everyone of closeness. It forces the child to live with the insecurity of never knowing for sure whether his father loves him.

But let's be fair to fathers. Most of us are not unaffectionate because we are cold, unloving people. Mother is right when she assures the child of his father's love. Father cares, but finds it difficult to show he cares because of irrational fears.

Men think of touching primarily in terms of sexual intercourse. Showing love through touching, kissing, hugging is uncomfortable for many men. One of the most encouraging developments among younger men is the acceptance of physical contact and hugging of friends (male and female). But for the average man, unfortunately, touch is associated with only two contexts: sex and aggressive contact such as sports or fighting. Perhaps this explains why the physical contact fathers have most often with their children involves roughhousing.

Men fear the possibility of becoming sexually aroused, so they avoid contact with their children. Many fathers stop being affectionate with their sons after age five or six for fear such behavior might be construed as being homosexual or might influence their sons to become homosexual. Similarly, they stop affection with their daughters (usually before puberty) for fear of appearing to be "dirty old men."

One of the father's greatest fears is getting an erection while playing with or being affectionate with his child. He worries this indicates something perverse or unnatural. Erection is usually a sign of sexual arousal, but sometimes it has no sexual connotation. Physiologically, high degrees of nonerotic excitement will elicit vascular responses, including erections. These stimuli can include anticipation of a competitive athletic event, excitement mixed with anxiety about going into combat, positive anticipation of receiving an award or bonus, as well as the enjoyment of playing with your child. An erection from a father-child interaction does not mean the father feels sexual toward his child. Even if the man's worst fears come true and the child notices the erection and comments on it, it can be explained as a natural reaction to enjoyable contact.

We want to make the point very clearly that sex educators and therapists are opposed to abusive sexual touching, exhibitionism, and voyeurism. Sexual contact has no place in a parent-child relationship. There are strong cultural taboos (not the mention legal ones) against inappropriate sexual touching. Child sex abuse and incest is a very negative experience, interfering with the child's psychological and sexual development. Inappropriate sexual touching is more likely to involve brothers, cousins, step-brothers, uncles, in-laws, and family friends rather than fathers. Although girls are most often victimized, in one-third of incidents boys are abused. Male children are less likely to reveal sexual abuse because they feel humiliated. There is a special stigma because it is a same sex incident (95 percent of abuse of girls and 90 percent of abuse of boys are perpetrated by males).

There is a clear distinction between genuine, healthy affection and sexual abuse. Affection is freely given and received, is non-genital, is clothed, can be talked about, and involves the genuine expression of warm feelings. Sexual abuse is coercive, for the man's sexual needs, involves inappropriate sexual viewing or touching, is secret, and creates confused and guilty feelings for the child.

HUSBAND-WIFE AFFECTION IN FRONT OF CHILDREN

Many men feel self-conscious about being affectionate with their spouse in the presence of their children. Again, the stereotypic intercourse-directed view of touch is to blame. If a kiss or hug is thought of as a prelude to intercourse, then a man will feel self-conscious about his children seeing them being affectionate. If, however, he thinks of affection as a normal way of showing love and caring, he is free to express himself. Being comfortable giving and receiving affection outside the bedroom is very important, not only for ourselves but for our children. If affection is a common occurrence between parents, the child learns it is a normal part of marriage.

Certain writers have taken the extreme view that none of a couple's interactions, including intercourse, ought to be kept private from their children. Such a total lack of restriction on sexual expression does a child harm. Children need to understand a sexual relationship is intimate and private. Sensual and/or sexual behavior between parents makes children uncomfortable. Children whose parents prided themselves on being sexually liberated will tell you what a burden it was to have this imposed on them. With sex, just as with material luxuries, it is possible to go overboard in trying to give your kids the things you never had. Establish rules of privacy that work both ways. Allow children a reasonable degree of privacy, and let them know parents need private couple time.

Harold and Susan

One couple we know have three children—ages six, nine, and eleven. After dinner, Harold and Susan spend a few minutes over coffee talking. During this time the children know their parents are not to be disturbed, so they play or do homework. If the telephone rings, they answer it and take messages.

A second guideline concerns the time Harold and Susan spend in their bedroom. When the door is open, the children come and go freely. When it is closed and locked, however, they know their parents are not to be disturbed except for emergencies. The children, naturally, have expressed curiosity about what goes on behind the locked bedroom door. Harold and Susan tell the children that while they love and enjoy being with them, they need time together. When the bedroom door is locked, they may be talking, taking a nap, making love or simply sharing couple time away from the hustle and bustle. The children accept this, although they giggle and make jokes. If a husband and wife are going to be effective parents, they need time as a couple. The most important bond in a family is the husband-wife bond; if that is attended to and reinforced it makes raising children easier. It is good for children to be aware their parents are also a husband and wife.

CHILDREN'S SEXUAL EXPLORATION

An important part of raising sexually healthy children is for parents to let children explore and touch their bodies. Parents need to feel comfortable allowing the young child to touch his genitals rather than slapping his hands and telling him it's bad or unclean. By age three or four, parents explain self-exploration is healthy and acceptable, but should occur in private rather than in public. Let the child know his body is good and it is okay to touch, but there is an appropriate time and place to do so.

The old folk tale was if a male child touched his penis "excessively" there would be terrible consequences. Since no one adequately defined excessive, the child was punished whenever he touched himself. If the child is not allowed to explore and touch, he gets the message there is something bad or dirty about his body and/or genitals.

It is natural for children to engage in sex play. "Playing doctor" or "playing house" are common activities—expressions of normal curiosity. This takes place between children of the same sex as well as children of the opposite sex, as well as among siblings. It is not a sign of promiscuity, incest, or homosexuality. The time to be concerned is if the activity becomes exploitative, aggressive, or involves significant (five years or more) age differences. Explorative sex play is normal. When the parent overreacts, the child is left with the message that touching is bad or disgusting. A healthier approach is to accept the activity and interfere only when it appears forced, coercive or becomes the dominant form of play. The child learns there is a time and place for sexual play; not in public, not as a dominant activity, and not in an aggressive or exploitative manner.

PARENT-CHILD SEXUAL COMMUNICATION

It is traditional for sexual information to be conveyed through talks between father and son or mother and daughter, but there is no reason why this rigid same-sex rule should be the only form of sexual communication. It makes a great deal of sense to have family sexuality discussions. Sexuality is a normal, good part of life rather than something to be whispered about in private. Sex education begins early in the child's life, with the parent teaching him proper names for his genitals. The child learns to be comfortable with *penis* and *vulva*, rather than euphemisms such as *whatsit* or *down there* or *my thing*.

How much information should the child be given? The best policy is to let the child's curiosity guide you. This allows the child to pace himself in terms of what he wants to know and is able to understand. If you respond in a positive and open manner, he gets the message sex is something that is okay to talk about, and he is free to ask again. Parents should not feel that because their five-year-old asks where babies come from, they have to tell him everything from contraception to homosexuality. Give the child the information he is seeking in words that make sense to him. Establish yourself as an "askable parent."

Comprehensive sex education is a combination of formal teaching provided by school, value-oriented approaches provided by religious groups, combined with an informal approach from parents. The parent might want to buy (or borrow from the library) a sexuality book written for your child's age. Instead of handing the book to the child, telling him to read it, and asking if he has any questions, try an approach that allows you to interact on a personal level. First read the book yourself or read it with your child. Point out parts you find particularly interesting or tell him about a misconception you had at his age. Rather than a question-and-answer format, the talk is a sharing process where you impart not only information but also feelings, attitudes, values, and experiences. If this pattern is established early, it makes later discussions about sex more comfortable, as well as frank and honest, especially important in the adolescent years. Discussions about sex can involve three-way conversations with both mother and father. Family meetings including both female and male children further increase the range of discussion.

SEXUAL COMMUNICATION WITH ADOLESCENTS

Being the parent of an adolescent is quite different from being the parent of a child. Adolescence can be a difficult and stressful period. Physical and psychological changes are rapid and profound. Within the space of a few years, he must adjust to a whole different set of needs, expectations, and responsibilities. Many societies, recognizing this transition is both difficult and highly significant, mark it with an initiation ceremony or rite of passage.

In our society, there is no event that signals the transition from child to adult. A father can play a significant part in easing the stress encountered by his adolescent son or daughter.

An adolescent is in the process of becoming a self-directing and autonomous individual capable of making his own decisions. A parent cannot hope to exert the same control over the adolescent as he did when the child was younger.

An adolescent must learn to make healthy decisions. One of the most important lessons is that actions have consequences. He and only he can be accountable for what he does. A parent should neither play the role of the tyrant, expecting to maintain iron control nor feel guilty when the adolescent makes mistakes. In either case, the parent would be performing a disservice by impeding the adolescent's process of maturation.

At the same time, a parent must be aware an adolescent is very much in need of support and guidance. An adolescent's first tentative entry into the world of adult freedom and responsibility may be exciting, but also confusing and frightening (for the adolescent as well as the parent). The adolescent needs to be aware of the parents' values and views about masturbation, dating, petting, contraception, premarital intercourse, and sexually transmitted diseases. The parent should be aware sexual behavior which is clearly inappropriate for a thirteen-year-old might be acceptable for a seventeen-year-old. The parents must make a distinction for themselves (as well as the adolescent) about the kind of behavior they will tolerate, even if they do not approve of it, and the behavior they will not tolerate. For example, some parents accept their eighteen-year-old son is having intercourse, but will not accept intercourse taking place in their home. Another example is the parent insisting the adolescent use condoms to protect against STDs/HIV, although the parent prefers he would not engage in intercourse until age 21.

The adolescent needs assurance both his parents—mother *and* father—will support and accept him. In the traditional pattern, it is the mother the child can count on to be accepting and comfort him when he gets into trouble, while the father plays the role of the stern disciplinarian. But there is no reason why a father should be less supportive than a mother. An adolescent needs support from both parents.

CLOSING THOUGHTS

It seems odd that children, the living evidence of their parents' sexuality, should be raised in such a way that the knowledge of sexuality is kept from them for as long as possible. Sexuality is not something that is conferred on a person at maturity like a driver's license or the right to vote. It is with us from the time we are born and, like our other natural faculties, needs to be developed. Don't deny your child the benefit of having a father as a positive role model, and don't deny yourself the opportunity to be a sex educator for your children.

12

SEX AND THE AGING MALE

How difficult is it for you to picture your parents making love? What about your grandparents? How would you feel about seeing a picture of a seventy-year-old woman as the centerfold of *Playboy?* Or a nude man in his seventies as the centerfold of *Playgirl?* Are you turned off by these images? If so, you share the dominant tendency in our society to deny the sexuality of older people. Where sex is concerned, we are youth chauvinists.

Our culture considers itself sexually liberated, but this does not extend to people over 60. Yes, sex has become more open, but only for that segment of the population between adolescence and the middle years of adulthood. For those above this chronological boundary, sexuality is not supposed to be important. It is assumed older people are less capable of sexual feelings, less interested in sexual expression. Men over 60 are considered "over the hill" and expected to lapse uncomplainingly into a peaceful, nonerotic state, free of sexual thoughts, fantasies, and desire.

In fact, we are sexual people from the day we are born to the day we die. Men (and women) in their sixties, seventies, eighties, and beyond can and do have sexual desire, enjoy sexual fantasies, experience sexual arousal, have intercourse, and are orgasmic. While a man's sexual responses change as he grows older, the aging man in good health is capable of sexual pleasure and functioning, being an involved partner, and is able to enjoy a variety of sexual activities, including intercourse. As a man grows older, sex is different from his younger days, but not less enjoyable. Older men are not high-frequency sexual athletes, but can be satisfying lovers.

THE NEGATIVE INFLUENCE OF AGEIST ATTITUDES

But if older men are capable of sexual functioning, why do so many give up on sex as they enter their fifties, sixties, and seventies? The answer is negative cultural conditioning and unrealistic, self-defeating expectations. Our society has not included sexuality as part of the "role" elderly people are supposed to assume. This is not true of other cultures, where it is considered natural for older people to show an interest in sexuality and lead active and fulfilling sex lives. Our society associates sexuality primarily with adolescents and young adults and sees sexual enjoyment as inappropriate for those over 60.

The double standard favors younger males, but subverts middle-aged and older men. Male sexual socialization for adolescents and young adults views arousal as easy, automatic, and predictable. Most important, males learn to function autonomously. They need nothing from the partner, other than her acquiescence. This expectation subverts sexual functioning in the 40s and 50s, and is absolutely poisonous for male sexual functioning after 60. The prescription of intimacy, nondemand pleasuring, and eroticism reaches its fruition with aging. It's especially important for the couple to be intimate sexual friends who accept a variable, flexible sexual style.

Only rarely is the sexuality of older persons presented in a sensitive, accepting manner by the media. More often, those over 60 who express sexual interest are assumed to be "dirty old men" or "perverts." Faced with such opposition, it is understandable that a large number of men give up and become resigned to a nonsexual existence. When couples stop having sex, in 90 percent of the cases, it is the man's decision.

Unfortunately, physicians, the very people men rely on for information about aging, share the false idea that sex probably will end in the sixties. But they are only reflecting our society's misconceptions. Many doctors were trained when there were no sexuality courses in medical schools, and may be unfamiliar with recent scientific findings about sex and aging. It is not uncommon to find older men discouraged from pursuing an active sex life or being told they must accept the loss of sexual desire and functioning. Some doctors, along with most laymen, think sexual dysfunction is a natural part of the aging process. But it's not.

Feeling unsure about their right to sexual feelings, older men block sexual thoughts and fantasies because they worry these are wrong or unnatural. As a result of this self-imposed mental censorship, men repress sexual desire and feelings. Others, while remaining in touch with their sexual feelings, become convinced they are no longer capable of acting upon them. If a man believes or fears he cannot get an erection, this becomes a self-fulfilling prophecy. The experience of erectile dysfunction reinforces the belief he is no longer a sexual man, and he resigns himself to a nonsexual life.

NORMAL CHANGES WITH AGING

There is no reason why an older man should stop being sexually active. Sexual functioning does not cease with age. Studies show healthy men, no matter what their age and whether or not they are active sexually, continue to have erections during sleep. If a man gets an erection in his sleep, he can have an erection with a partner. He is able to enjoy sexual activity, including, but not limited to, intercourse. There is no more reason for a man to lose his ability to have sex than for him to lose the ability to engage in any other natural function. A man of seventy cannot run as fast as he could when he was twenty, but he is able to enjoy a brisk walk. Similarly, an older man will not respond as rapidly to sexual stimulation or ejaculate as frequently, but can enjoy sex on a regular basis. The crucial attitude is he deserves sexual pleasure. Sexuality is part of life. As long as he is alive, a man has a right to be sexual and find pleasure with touching and eroticism.

A major reason older men become discouraged is they are not aware of the sexual changes that gradually occur as a result of aging. If he doesn't understand these, he is liable to misinterpret changes as a sign he is losing sexual capability. Consequently, he becomes anxious about his erotic capacity. He either avoids sex altogether or becomes so anxious about performing that sex is no longer enjoyable. There is no reason to fall into this trap. A man who is aware what to expect (and shares this knowledge with his partner), can derive as much enjoyment from sex as ever—in some ways, even more.

When in his teens and twenties, the man had "automatic" erections and functioned autonomously (i.e., he needed nothing from the woman in order to feel desire, achieve erection, and reach orgasm). However, most men in their forties, and almost all men by their sixties, need for sex to be a shared, cooperative, interactive process. The woman's active involvement and pleasure is integral to his enjoyment and functioning. All the lessons on respectful, cooperative male-female intimacy, enjoyment of nondemand pleasuring, and need for erotic stimulation come to fruition during the aging process. The man who is aware of and accepting of these concepts before age sixty will to make a positive transition to sex and aging.

A change which commonly occurs is a decrease in the need for ejaculation at each sexual experience. This, like most sexual changes, is a gradual process which occurs before 60, although there is a great deal of variation from one individual to another. Men find they do not need to ejaculate each time they have intercourse even though they are aroused and are enjoying the sexual experience.[9] If a man does not feel the desire on a particular occasion, he should not try to force ejaculation, just enjoy the pleasurable sensations. Vasocongestion of the testicles during arousal is not pronounced in older men, so there will not be a problem with "blue balls" as a result of not ejaculating.

This decrease in the urge for ejaculation is natural, not to be confused with ejaculatory inhibition. The aging man can accept this change and not try to force ejaculation when he has no need or desire. There are other differences to be aware of. Ejaculation lasts a shorter time, his penis contracts fewer times, semen comes out less forcefully, and less semen is ejaculated. Instead of ejaculation being a two-step process, consisting of the point of ejaculatory inevitability followed by ejaculation, it is a single-stage process. With aging, sex becomes less ejaculation oriented but not less pleasure oriented.

Some men report experiencing an orgasm without ejaculating. Other men say they did not have an orgasm but did enjoy the sexual experience. Some report experiencing an intensity of pleasure equivalent to orgasm.

Another difference is once he's ejaculated, his penis becomes flaccid much faster than in earlier years. This causes the man to fear he is losing his sexual powers and worry he may not be able to achieve an erection. This fear is confused with the fact that he experiences a longer refractory period. Following ejaculation, he will not be able to achieve another erection for a period varying from several hours to a full day, while as a young man he could get a second erection in an hour or less. However, this is not a reason for performance anxiety. His sexual responses are slowing, but this doesn't mean they are about to stop. If he accepts the altered sexual pace that comes with aging, he will find sex satisfying. The adage that as one ages he is less of a sexual athlete, but more a sensuous lover, is true.

One advantage of the less urgent need to ejaculate is he exceeds the younger man in ejaculatory control. This greater control can enhance sexual enjoyment, including intercourse, for both people. As sex becomes less ejaculation oriented, he is able to relax and be receptive to the myriad, subtle, whole-body sensations of lovemaking. As his ability to both give and receive pleasure increases, he becomes a more sensitive lover.

Along with the lessened need for ejaculation, the process of sexual arousal slows. While a younger man may require only seconds of stimulation before getting an erection, an older man may need several minutes or more. In addition, he needs direct penile stimulation to become fully aroused. A young man may get an erection just from thinking about sex or seeing his partner's nude body. With older men, it is necessary for the partner to use stroking, oral, or rubbing stimulation. Once achieved, his erection is not as full as in earlier days. The woman can take the initiative and guide intromission. He does not need a completely firm erection to enjoy eroticism and intercourse. Arousal builds with thrusting. Her receptivity and responsivity increases his arousal.

FEMALE CHANGES

A woman's sexual responses change as she grows older. For women, menopause (which is typically a two-year process occurring between ages forty-five and fifty-five) serves as a clear milestone of physical change. Male changes are gradual and less obvious. In addition to the cessation of menstruation, the vagina becomes smaller and the vaginal walls thinner and less elastic. The breasts and clitoris decrease in size and firmness. These changes do not negatively affect her responsiveness to sexual stimulation. The woman's response pattern is much the same as when she was younger, but slower. Changes in female sexual response are less dramatic than for males.

It will take the older woman longer to become lubricated, and the amount of lubrication will not be as great as when she was younger. Many couples find it helpful to use a sterile lubricant such Astroglide, abalone lotion, K-Y Jelly or a nonallergenic lotion such as baby oil, Lubriderm, or a nice smelling lotion from Crabtree and Evelyn, all available without a prescription. Saliva can serve as an excellent and perfectly safe lubricant.

A common fear is menopause will put an end to the woman's sexual desire. Hysterectomy (the surgical removal of the uterus) is thought to be the death knell for a woman's sexuality. Neither of these beliefs is valid. In fact, many women feel freer and more sexual because they no longer worry about an unwanted pregnancy. The more the woman (and man) know about menopause and female aging the less likely it will have a negative effect on sexual expression. In fact, female arousal is easier and more predictable than male arousal. Her arousal can facilitate his arousal.

POSITIVE FACTORS IN THE AGING PROCESS

Aging brings changes in the sexual functioning of both men and women. These changes are not indications a person's sex life is over, but entering a new phase, taking on a new style. Sex between older people tends to be slower, gentler, and most importantly, more intimate and interactive. He can enjoy experiencing and giving pleasure rather than turning in a stellar performance. He needs to feel comfortable requesting stimulation, especially erotic scenarios and manual or oral penile stimulation he finds most arousing.

It helps if he can learn to appreciate other aspects of sex besides intercourse and orgasm—open himself to the limitless possibilities of increased sensual awareness, pleasuring, and eroticism. He can utilize the guidelines presented throughout this book in order to maintain a satisfying sex life. He must learn, if he has not already done so, to be a sensuous lover rather than an athletic performer. Changes in his body facilitate this adjustment, provided he accepts them. But if he fights the course of nature, he is bound to lose. Being a sexual man of seventy is different from being a sexual man of twenty. But the essence of sexuality—pleasure and sharing—remains central.

Aging is not an illness; it's a natural physiological process. The more a man takes care of himself, eats well, maintains a healthy sleep pattern, exercises regularly, does not smoke, if he drinks does so in moderation, and stays in good health, the better his body will adjust to aging and the better his sexual functioning will be. One mistake men make is to assume frequent sexual contacts wear them out or use up their sexual capability. If he is unable to get an erection or ejaculate on a particular occasion, he avoids sex for a month to give himself a rest. This is the wrong approach. You do not need a rest from sex. What you need are broad-based sensual and sexual experiences on a regular basis.

The idea a man only has a certain number of ejaculations and when they are used up his sex life is over is false. In fact, the more regular his sexual expression, the easier it is to continue sexual functioning. A popular phrase "Use it or lose it," is true. A regular rhythm of sexual expression facilitates sexual functioning. By continuing to be affectionate and sensual, enjoying pleasuring and eroticism, having intercourse and ejaculating regularly, he maintains the self-confidence needed for a vital sex life.

SEXUALITY AND ILLNESS

Of course, not all men are in good physical health. Certain diseases (for instance, cancer, diabetes, multiple sclerosis, and kidney dysfunction) can interfere with sexual functioning. In fact, any illness (as well as side effects of medication) can inhibit sexual activity, but does not end it. Too often, men who have prostate surgery, a heart attack, stroke, lung disease, cancer, diabetes, and other illnesses assume they can no longer be sexually active. If you have an illness, gain as full an understanding of it as possible, including its effect on your sexuality. Consult your physician, accompanied by your wife if possible, and explain that sex is an important part of your life. You want to know what changes to make in your sexual activities, if any. Remember, however, many physicians have little training in sexuality and may not be comfortable or competent discussing sexual concerns and problems.

If you are not satisfied with the advice of your physician, the next step would be to consult a physician with a subspecialty in sexual medicine. He or she will explain how sexual functioning may be affected by the illness or medications you are taking. If you have an illness that places limitations on your sex life, it is best to discuss these problems openly with your partner. Explore feelings and communicate about changes in the sexual relationship. Even in cases where intercourse may be limited or impossible (chronic diabetes, hypertension, or vascular disorders) there are other ways to share pleasurable, sensual, and sexual experiences. These include manual stimulation, giving and receiving oral stimulation, hugging, massage, and nondemand pleasuring. You could explore medical interventions such as injections, external pump, prostheses or sexual medications.

While a disease or medications might limit a man's ability to have erections, his ability to have orgasms is usually unimpaired. Thus, it can be quite satisfying to continue sensual and sexual interactions. Too many couples are willing to give up sex entirely when illness or physical incapacity strikes. As a culture, we think of sex as for the young, the strong, and the healthy. In fact, sexual pleasure is one of the basic constants of life. It is available to both the young and old, the healthy and the not so healthy. You need not give up on sex or tell your partner your sexual days are over. Affection, touching, and intimacy make life enjoyable. A person is entitled to be sexual, whatever his age or physical condition.

In a small number of older men, a decrease in testosterone affects their sexual desire. These men can derive great benefit from consulting an endocrinologist or urologist and receiving testosterone replacement therapy.

Couples with a sexual dysfunction sometimes use their age as an excuse to avoid seeking treatment. Their fear that they're "too old" for sex is unjustified since therapists report a higher success rate with couples in their sixties and seventies than with younger couples. Success in sex therapy depends on the couple's commitment, their ability to discuss feelings and sexual requests, desire for touching and eroticism, and flexibility in utilizing pleasuring and erotic techniques, not on how old they are.

Karl and Trudy

Karl and Trudy were in their mid-seventies when they saw Barry for sex therapy. Karl had owned a small chemical plant and was actively involved in the business until age 68. He decided to spend the rest of his life enjoying hobbies and activities he didn't have time for while working. So, he sold that business and retired. The transition from active businessman to retirement was difficult for Karl. This is not unusual—the two most common problems for retired males are depression and alcoholism (both of which have negative effects on sexual functioning). The lack of self-respect manifested itself as an erection problem. Karl and Trudy had resigned themselves to a life without sex until Trudy confided the problem to their minister. He suggested they consult a sex therapist.

Once they accepted the idea that it was not normal for sexual functioning to stop, Karl and Trudy began to make progress. Nondemand pleasuring exercises were initiated. Trudy was very pleased with the reintroduction of intimacy, touching, and pleasuring. Karl's interest and desire rebounded, partly in reaction to Trudy's. After six weeks they reintroduced eroticism and intercourse. Their lovemaking was more frequent and pleasurable than in the past twenty years. Just as important, Karl made changes in how he structured his time. He made a positive adjustment to retirement, which enhanced his psychological and sexual well-being.

OLDER, SINGLE MALES

So far, we have been discussing married men. What about the man who is widowed or divorced? While many men remarry and others have dating partners, a good number feel sexual urges yet do not have a partner. One valid outlet is masturbation. Our culture views masturbation as appropriate mainly for boys and young men. Masturbation can be an important and healthy means of sexual expression for the older man as well. No one should feel guilty about masturbation. Many older men (including well-functioning married men) masturbate, which is just as normal as for young men.

It is quite common for older men to remarry. Because women have eight years greater life expectancy, the number of women in proportion to men increases steadily with age. An older man who wishes to remarry finds no shortage of available partners. However, the man makes the mistake of seeing his second marriage as a replacement for the first one. In establishing an emotional and sexual relationship, it is important to view this as new and unique, don't compare it with the first marriage. Be aware of the preferences and feelings of the new spouse and communicate your needs and desires. Don't assume that what worked in the last relationship will work in this one. You need to explore, be spontaneous, and communicate so you establish a satisfying emotional and sexual bond.

CLOSING THOUGHTS

The attempt to set an age limit on sexuality is both unrealistic and unjust. We never outgrow sex, nor does a healthy man (or woman) lose his desire for intimacy, touching, eroticism and sexuality. Even where physical disability or illness is present, the need for sensual and sexual expression remains, which can be acknowledged and acted upon. The couple who enjoy sexuality in old age are extremely fortunate. They should not feel self-conscious about their continuing desire for each other. They can take pride in keeping their relationship vital and taking full advantage of it. If they understand and accept the unique characteristics of sexuality in the later years, they will find their sexual relationship becoming more sensitive, sharing, tender, and enjoyable.

13
REGAINING SEXUAL DESIRE

Inhibited sexual desire (ISD) is the most common complaint which brings couples to sex therapy. But isn't sexual desire a problem solely for women? In our macho culture, where a "real man wants to have sex with any woman, any time, and in any situation" can there be a problem with male desire? The traditional view is that a man, especially a young man, is controlled by his penis: "A hard cock has no conscience."

The reality is ISD occurs on occasion for almost every man. For ten to fifteen percent of men it is a chronic problem, becoming more frequent and severe with age.[10] It's easier to admit to a performance dysfunction (early ejaculation, erectile dysfunction, ejaculatory inhibition) than to a lack of sexual desire. Desire is viewed as a natural characteristic of male sexuality, a measure of masculinity. Embarrassment about having a desire problem is so great that men resist psychotherapy or sex therapy. If he is coerced into therapy by his partner, his goal is to minimize the problem and get out of treatment as quickly as possible.

Sexual desire problems are more prevalent than believed. If you use an arbitrary definition of being sexual less than 10 times a year, approximately 20 percent of married couples and 35 percent of nonmarried couples who've been together more than two years have a nonsexual relationship.[11] Men blame desire problems on outside sources (job, spouse's weight, lack of time, sex becoming routine). They want a "magic pill" or an outside source (a twenty-year-old sexy woman) to regain desire. It's as if desire isn't an integral part of the man, but comes from external sources.

INHIBITIONS THAT BLOCK SEXUAL DESIRE

The key element in sexual desire is anticipation. Ideally, the man feels he deserves sexual pleasure and anticipates the sexual experience. Desire is affected by physical factors including illness, side effects of medication, drug or alcohol abuse, low testosterone, fatigue or stress, and poor health habits. Physical factors can be evaluated during a general medical exam by your internist, but these are usually not the prime factor in ISD. The man hopes the problem is medical so he can take a pill and sexual desire will magically return to a robust state. If there is no specific medical diagnosis and treatment (which is true for the great majority of cases), he needs to examine psychological, relational, and situational causes. Even when there are medical factors which can be treated, he still needs to address these issues.

The best way to understand the problem is by becoming aware of "inhibitions" that block anticipation, thus the term *inhibited sexual desire, ISD*. Primary ISD means the man has never had desire for partner sex. This is rare, although more common among women since our culture gives less permission for women to value and express their sexuality. Approximately 33 percent of women experience ISD, half is primary and half secondary. Common causes for primary ISD among men are a compulsive masturbatory technique or fantasy (usually a fetish arousal pattern), trauma caused by sexual or physical abuse, conflict regarding sexual orientation, or negative attitudes toward sex, often governed by rigid religious beliefs or an antisex family environment.

Far more common is secondary ISD which affects 15 percent of men, and 30 percent of men over fifty. In fact, one of the most thought-provoking statistics is when couples stop having sex, in over ninety percent of the cases it is the man's decision. This is conveyed indirectly and nonverbally. Sex has become more of a chore or source of frustration than a pleasure, and he adopts an avoidance strategy.

The most common cause for secondary ISD is sexual dysfunction, i.e., erectile problems and to a lesser extent orgasm problems. The dysfunction sets the stage for a cycle of negative anticipation, tense or disappointing sexual experiences, followed by increasingly long periods of avoidance. As the man's sense of frustration and failure increases, his anticipation and desire decreases, and he avoids sexual thoughts or interactions.

Another cause of ISD is the man who wants to function "automatically" (needing nothing from his partner). As he ages or sex falls into a mechanical routine, he discovers automatic functioning is no longer possible. Rather than communicating this and developing an intimate, interactive sexual relationship, he withdraws, hoping "horniness" will develop from deprivation. This is a self-defeating strategy since a key element in sexual desire is a regular rhythm of sexual expression. For example, testosterone increases after orgasm. The nonsexual pattern leads to increased avoidance and decreased desire. Thus, the man sets himself (and his relationship) on a path of minimal or nonexistent sexual activity.

A third cause is negative emotions, especially anxiety, depression, or anger. Sexuality is associated with positive emotions and motivations; negative emotions can and do inhibit desire. Negative emotions, both sexual and nonsexual, need to be dealt with directly so they don't subvert sexuality. Anxiety is the problem easiest to treat. Sex therapy focuses on reducing anticipatory and performance anxiety. Treatment involves gradually approaching the sexual inhibition and regaining sexual comfort and confidence. Lowered sexual desire can be a sign of depression. Men tend to deny feeling depressed and go on with their routines at work and home, but with minimal involvement and pleasure. Males prefer antidepressant medication rather than examining and changing the psychological, relational, and situational factors that cause and maintain their depression (the strategy Barry strongly advises). Antidepressant drugs can have negative effects on sexual functioning, especially ability to be orgasmic and feel desire. The question is can the man's mood be lifted without these side effects. Anger is the most difficult emotion to deal with because males stubbornly hang on to their anger. Being "right" and winning the angry power struggle becomes more important than resuming the sexual relationship. Anger usually involves nonsexual issues, but it poisons the sexual relationship. The longer the anger is held and the more it is expressed through verbal abuse and/or physical violence, the more detrimental to sexual desire (this is also true for women). The man and couple need to learn to express angry feelings in nondestructive ways, explore the hurt behind the anger, problem-solve to resolve the conflict, and reach agreements both people can live with. Nonsexual anger needs to be dealt with outside the bedroom rather than sex being the battleground.

Alcohol and drug abuse (especially cocaine and barbiturates) have long-term negative effects on sexual desire. This is paradoxical, since reducing sexual inhibitions was one of the supposed functions of alcohol. Cocaine had been touted as the "perfect aphrodisiac." In truth, anything which depresses the central nervous system (especially more than 3 drinks or chronic drug abuse) inhibits sexual expression. Drug and alcohol abuse have a number of physical and psychological effects which subvert sexual desire. Cigarette smoking also has negative sexual effects because it interferes with vascular functioning. Desire is not going to be revitalized until the substance abuse is resolved.

Relationship problems are a major cause of ISD. Men have a tendency to take their marriage for granted and allow it to become dull and stagnant. Relationships need attention to thrive. It's easy to fall into the trap of being frustrated with the spouse and marriage. Instead of marriage being a growth-enhancing, positive influence, the relationship degenerates into a bitter standoff. The marital bond needs to be revitalized, which facilitates sexual desire. It is not a simple matter of cause and effect, but a reciprocal relationship between emotional and sexual intimacy.

There are numerous possible causes of ISD—including acute or chronic illness, sexual phobias or aversions, fear of pregnancy, emotional alienation, negative attitudes toward sexuality, stress from children or jobs, lack of time or privacy. The man and couple need to be honest in identifying the factors that block sexual desire and instituting a plan for change. ISD is a problem that responds better to professional therapy rather than self-help approaches because of its multicausal, multidimensional nature. The role of the therapist is to keep the couple motivated and focused so they can revitalize sexual desire.

Jonathon and Marie

Regaining sexual desire is a function of the man's increasing awareness, assuming responsibility for his sexuality, and working with his partner to develop a functional and satisfying sexual style. Jonathon presents a good illustration of this complex, yet achievable, process. Jonathon is a forty-three-year-old consulting engineer married 17 years to Marie. They had allowed sexuality to slip away in the past five years beginning when Jonathon had difficulty maintaining an erection during intercourse. On some occasions he experienced ejaculatory inhibition and other times early ejaculation. Rather than discussing this and working with Marie to develop comfortable, arousing and erotic sexual scenarios, he became distant emotionally and sexually.

The sexual dysfunction left him vulnerable to an affair with his partner's secretary. The affair was very exciting and sexually fulfilling. Sexual novelty and illicitness along with the psychological charge from feeling desired and attractive carried Jonathon for three months. However, things started collapsing like a house of cards. His business partner was infuriated with Jonathon since the secretary had been doing marginal work and now her work was unsatisfactory. Jonathon's own work was suffering, and clients were complaining to other partners. The affair became a major source of office gossip, and colleagues were saying very unkind things behind his back. Someone made an anonymous phone call to Marie, who confronted Jonathon. She felt hurt, confusion, and anger. Jonathon denied everything, which only made matters worse. The breakup of the affair extended over six months (affairs are much easier to get into than out of). By this time Jonathon was experiencing sexual dysfunction both in his marriage and in the affair. As the debris settled, he withdrew emotionally and sexually. Jonathon wanted to stay away from sex since it had caused so much pain and embarrassment. For the next two years, his sexual outlet was masturbation, which he put down as an adolescent behavior.

Jonathon was forced into therapy by a frustrated and angry Marie, who demanded they deal with the affair and their nonsexual marriage. To say he was a reluctant client is an understatement; he saw nothing in therapy for him except further embarrassment and failure. Negative motivation seldom promotes positive behavior. The first therapeutic task was to identify goals with Jonathon. He was encouraged to view his masturbation differently. Since he felt desire, was aroused, had an erection, and enjoyed orgasm, he was reassured everything was intact physiologically. Sex could be a source of pleasure and satisfaction. The next step was restructuring his thoughts toward Marie and marital sexuality. Marie could be his sexual friend rather than his harshest personal and sexual critic. Jonathon and Marie began a series of sensual and sexual exercises to rebuild comfort, attraction, and trust. Psychological issues concerning anger and resentment were dealt with in the therapy sessions. They made an upfront agreement not to engage in affairs and to discuss any potential high risk situation. Marie realized they'd treated their intimate relationship with benign neglect. The best prevention strategy was to reestablish a vital marital bond. Jonathon admitted he'd taken the easy way out by not dealing with Marie and opting for an affair. He committed to address psychological conflicts and sexual problems directly, and not avoid.

Jonathon came to enjoy the nondemand pleasuring sessions, they added a new dimension to his life and revitalized marital intimacy. Rather than sex being a drain on his self-esteem, it became an energizing force, a way to share pleasure, reduce frustration, and build intimacy. Jonathon and Marie established bridges to sexual desire and a variable, flexible sexual style which allowed them to enjoy a variety of pleasurable and erotic sexual scenarios.

REGAINING SEXUAL DESIRE

In regaining sexual desire and rebuilding sexual anticipation, the man needs to be aware of and responsible for changing his sexual attitudes, behavior, and feelings. First is a commitment to rebuild sexual self-esteem and honestly assess (rather than avoid, deny, or minimize) elements that block sexual desire. He can do this on his own, with a therapist, or with his partner, but he needs to be honest in identifying inhibitions and developing a plan.

Self-exploration/masturbation exercises accompanied by experimentation with sexual fantasies are the most powerful individual intervention. This allows the man to regain confidence in a situation where he exerts control. In addition, it permits him to identify special turn-ons and arousal techniques. Additional individual interventions focus on changes in body image. These include stopping smoking or reducing drinking, beginning a weight-reduction or exercise program, practicing better personal hygiene, dressing in an attractive manner.

Another individual change technique is to think out, talk out, write out, or fantasize about sexual scenarios which would enhance desire. Bridges to sexual desire are strategies and techniques to build connection, pleasure, and eroticism. Design two sexual scenarios that lead to erotic anticipation. What would the foreplay/pleasuring be like? How would intercourse be initiated, what position would you enjoy most, what kind of thrusting would you use? What forms of multiple stimulation during intercourse would increase eroticism? How would the afterplay/afterglow phase be played out? How can you enhance emotional and sexual satisfaction?

COUPLE ISSUES IN INHIBITED SEXUAL DESIRE

More than any other sexual difficulty, ISD involves the couple's relationship. The famous story in sex therapy is the woman who came to a sex therapy clinic with her second husband. The problem was sexual desire. The therapist recalled the woman had been at the clinic five years before with her first husband. The problem had been he wanted to be sexual twice a day and she wanted to be sexual twice a week. With her second husband, she still wanted to be sexual twice a week, but he only desired to be sexual once a month. Sexual desire problems are best conceptualized as a discrepancy in expectations and feelings. There is not a ''right'' or ''normal'' number of times to have intercourse. Couples need to develop their style of being sexual—there is not ''one right'' style or frequency. The average range of intercourse frequency is from once every two weeks to three times a week. The couple have to find the mix of affectionate, sensual, erotic, and intercourse connection which fits their relationship. Sex therapy exercises provide guidelines to facilitate communication and experimentation. We encourage each couple to discuss what is comfortable and satisfying for them.

Sexual desire is the core of sexuality. Desire involves biological, psychological, relational, cultural, and situational factors. It can and does vary with individuals and couples. Desire can be facilitated and enhanced, as well as negated and subverted.

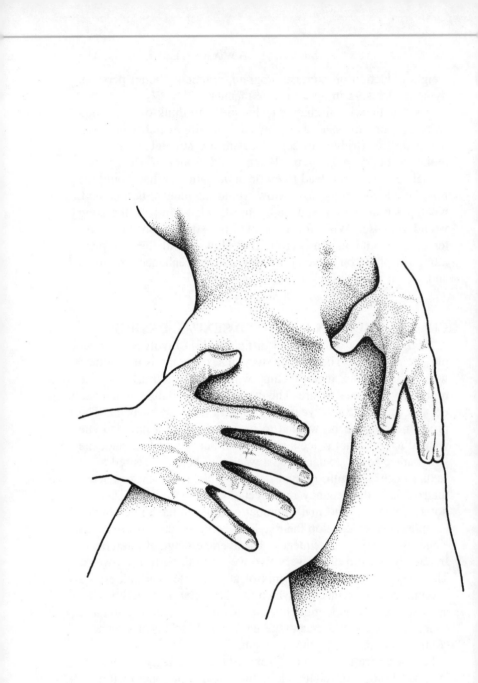

Holding, caressing and pleasuring build anticipation and pleasure.

ISD is best conceptualized as a couple problem. Building bridges to sexual desire is likewise best thought of as a couple process. This does not mean each bridge has to be mutual. Some strategies and techniques work better for one partner than the other.

Sexuality is a one-two combination. First, you are responsible for your sexuality, including desire. Second, intimate sexuality is about sharing, facilitating, encouraging, and supporting. It's not only normal, but preferable, for each spouse to have his/her bridges for desire. Having a multitude of ways to anticipate and initiate sexual experiences ensures that once the cycle of avoidance and the nonsexual marriage is broken, sexual desire will remain vital. It is healthy to have a variety of ways of emotionally and sexually connecting. A range of flexible bridges facilitates sexual intimacy. Choice, rather than obligation, enhances desire. When sex degenerates into "are we going to have intercourse or not?" the couple is in trouble. When one spouse demands intercourse and the other avoids pressure and coercion, the result is a power struggle and a nonsexual marriage.

A major cause of secondary ISD is taking the relationship for granted. If we put as little thought and energy into our businesses as we do into our marriages, there would be many bankrupt businesses. To maintain emotional intimacy and satisfying sexuality the couple needs to devote quality time, both inside and outside the bedroom.

Anger and lack of respect for your spouse subverts sexual desire. For sex to remain vital, you need to maintain a bond of respect, trust, and intimacy. Anger at one's spouse, whether for sexual or nonsexual reasons, festers and wears away at the marital bond. When the conflict is nonsexual, the couple is encouraged to deal with it directly rather than playing it out through sexual avoidance. If the anger revolves around a sexual issue (extramarital affairs, fertility problems, feeling sexually rejected, believing the spouse is sexually selfish, arguments over oral sex), the hurt feelings need to be addressed by talking outside the bedroom. Commit to resolving the sexual conflict.

Sex is often relegated to the last thing at night after taking care of the children, doing the dishes, watching endless TV, walking the dog. Good quality sex needs an awake, aware, involved couple. Sexuality has to assume a higher priority. Being open to sex in the morning or as a "nooner" on the weekend goes a long way toward restoring sexual desire.

Paul and Sylvia

Paul had been an ardent pursuer of Sylvia fourteen years earlier. At thirty-two, Paul felt ready to marry and was powerfully attracted to twenty-seven-year-old Sylvia. Paul had been offered a partnership in his law firm, this had taken the majority of his time and energy for the past seven years. Paul was energetic and goal-oriented, and this was transformed into an intense and passionate courtship. Sylvia reveled in the attention and happily entered into marriage. They had two daughters in five years, and much of their energy went into parenting. Paul was involved with his career, politics, golf, and parenting. Sex slipped into a Saturday-night routine. Sex was functional, but not creative or exciting. Sylvia became increasingly frustrated with Paul and their marriage. She resented how little time they spent as a couple, and how little affection (except for perfunctory hello/goodbye kisses) was displayed. Sylvia developed a reactive depression and reported no sexual desire. During the previous year, they had intercourse only three times. Paul's reaction was passive acceptance and a marked decrease in desire. This was a couple in trouble and headed for severe marital and sexual dysfunction.

To reverse this trend, Paul and Sylvia entered couples therapy. Revitalizing sexual desire was a primary goal. The first "homework exercise" was to restart an affectionate and sensuous relationship both inside and outside the bedroom. They took turns engaging in caressing and stroking in the bedroom with clothes on while verbalizing their feelings. Paul was cautioned not to make sex a goal-oriented work task, instead to be an active, involved partner in the process of giving and receiving pleasure. One night, they took the children to the in-laws' and instead of going to the movies returned home. They experimented with sensuous, nondemand touching in the nude while in the living room. To prevent interruptions they locked the doors and turned the answering machine on. To set a mood they put on their favorite music and used soft lighting. To enhance sensations they used a body lotion they had jointly chosen at Crabtree and Evelyn. These experiences made Paul and Sylvia aware of how much they were cheating themselves and each other by settling for a nonsexual marriage. Sensual touching reignited sexual anticipation and intimacy.

Another "homework exercise" focused on emotional and sexual attraction. Attraction is an ongoing process, building on the elements (physical, emotional, and interpersonal) you value in your partner. In our culture, myths about romantic love and "chemical" attraction abound. The reality is romantic love feelings seldom last more than a year or two. They are replaced by mature intimacy, where feelings of attraction are nurtured and anticipation reinforced by fulfilling sexual experiences.

Paul began by saying the things he found most attractive about Sylvia. This included her sparkling green eyes, her concern for their house and children, the way she looked at him when they kissed, her smell when she became sexually aroused. He was encouraged to spend as much time as he wanted acknowledging all the things that made her an attractive person. Sylvia actively listened and accepted the compliments, not shrugging them off or saying "Yes, but." Paul made two specific requests for change that would make Sylvia more attractive to him. Paul asked her to wear sexy clothing to bed—either a silky nightgown or his shirt with nothing else. He requested she tell him when she wanted to be sexual. Roles were reversed, and Sylvia had a chance to acknowledge Paul's attractiveness and make requests for change.

As sexual exercises continued, both experienced renewed anticipation, valuing their time as a couple, enjoying affection and pleasuring, and intercourse and orgasm again became a part of their marriage.

KEYS TO MAINTAINING SEXUAL DESIRE

When you get away from embarrassment and recriminations and see inhibited sexual desire as a couple problem, you are on the road to revitalizing your sexual bond. Instead of arguing about the past, focus on developing a functional and satisfying sexual style for the present and future. Touching can occur both inside and outside the bedroom. Not all touch can or should lead to intercourse. Rather than worry about the frequency of intercourse, enjoy the quality of your intimate relationship. Enjoy talking and laughing, sometimes planning sex and other times being spontaneous. Value affectionate, sensual, erotic, and intercourse touching. Especially important is establishing a rhythm of being sexual, at least once every other week. Reestablish the expectation that sex is a pleasurable and energizing part of your life. Emotional intimacy and flexibility in sensual and sexual expression is an excellent foundation for maintaining sexual desire.

14
LEARNING EJACULATORY CONTROL

Early (also called rapid or premature) ejaculation is the most common male sexual problem. Approximately three of ten men are early ejaculators. Until recently early ejaculation was viewed as a sign of masculinity, not a dysfunction. The traditional attitude was self-defeating, for the man as well as the couple's sexual relationship.

The great majority of men begin as early ejaculators. Among adolescent boys, masturbation is a secretive, hidden activity, haunted by guilt and fear of discovery. Adolescents try to reach orgasm as quickly as possible. In the so-called "circle jerk," when a group of adolescent boys masturbate in unison, the winner (viewed as most masculine) is the one who ejaculates the fastest and farthest. Male sexuality is dominated by performance pressures which subvert sexual self-esteem and couple intimacy.

This push toward rapid performance carries over to intercourse. Typically, a young man's first intercourse takes place in the back of a car in a hurried manner, on a sofa in the girl's house with the fear her parents may return at any moment, or with a prostitute who puts pressure on him to finish quickly so she can get on with business. These situations involve sexual excitement mixed with anxiety and a demand to perform rapidly. The young man is concerned with proving himself sexually rather than the pleasurable and erotic aspects of the experience. He associates sexual prowess with short, intense intercourse rather than giving and receiving pleasure. The vast majority of males reach orgasm very quickly in initial intercourse experiences. First intercourse involves high expectations, high excite-

189

ment, high anxiety, and little skill. In fact, many men ejaculate before intromission. This is the major cause of unsuccessful first intercourse, which occurs to one in four males. Sexual excitement and anxiety are closely associated. The outcome is a habit of early ejaculation.

MISUNDERSTANDINGS ABOUT EARLY EJACULATION

Although most men learn to slow down, enjoy their own and their partner's pleasure, and become comfortable and confident with sexual functioning, early ejaculation continues to be a problem for 30 percent of men.[12] Until recently, early ejaculation was not recognized as detrimental to the man or couple. When intercourse was seen primarily as a man's right and a woman's duty, he had little motivation to prolong sex. Since "nice" women were not expected to value sex, a man who could get the job done quickly was admired. If his wife found intercourse unpleasant or uncomfortable, she would urge him to "get done." This kind of thinking lingers to a pronounced degree even now, especially among men who don't realize women can enjoy eroticism and intercourse. Men generally, and early ejaculators particularly, are too fast and too rough in lovemaking. This hurried style is off-putting to women who desire sensual and slow pleasuring, creative and erotic stimulation, and prolonged and involving intercourse. Unfortunately, problems often become worse when the woman voices her dissatisfaction.

Misunderstandings about early ejaculation can create a great deal of tension. The woman feels he doesn't care about her sexual needs or her as a person. Instead of a shared, intimate experience, sex becomes a battleground. The man reacts in either of two ways, both destructive. The first is to become defensive and counterattack, telling his partner she is demanding and sex will be his way or he'll find a less critical partner. This leaves the woman stymied and resentful. The second self-defeating reaction is the man feels he is a sexual failure, apologizes, and becomes depressed. He avoids the source of his depression— sexual activity. When he does have sex, he tries to withhold ejaculation by biting his tongue, fixing his mind on anti-erotic thoughts, using a special anesthetizing cream on the tip of the penis, wearing two condoms. This reduces sexual pleasure, but does not increase ejaculatory control. He does not enjoy ejaculation because he is busy blaming himself for coming too quickly. Sex is not enjoyable, and he's vulnerable to developing an erection problem.

THE WOMAN'S ROLE IN DEALING WITH EJACULATORY CONTROL

Even men who recognize early ejaculation is a problem view the situation in a distorted and self-defeating light. They assume early ejaculation is detrimental only to the woman's enjoyment and prolonging intercourse is exclusively for her, so she can have an orgasm. The man mistakenly believes if he lasted longer she would automatically become orgasmic during intercourse. In fact, there needs to be more than just prolonged thrusting for women to reach climax. Surveys indicate the percentage of women who experience orgasm regularly during intercourse varies from one-fourth to half. Women enjoy the sexual experience, including intercourse, but most women find it easier to be orgasmic during nonintercourse sex (i.e., manual, oral, or rubbing stimulation).

Female orgasm does not occur automatically as a result of prolonged intercourse. One-third of women are regularly orgasmic, but never orgasmic during intercourse. Other women can be orgasmic during intercourse, but find being orgasmic through manual or oral stimulation easier and more predictable. Being nonorgasmic during intercourse is not a sexual dysfunction, it's a normal variation of female sexuality. Female arousal and orgasm is a matter of individual style and preference.

A woman who wishes to be orgasmic during intercourse will find it easier if her partner has good ejaculatory control and if they use multiple stimulation during intercourse. Most women who are orgasmic during intercourse do so with 4-7 minutes of thrusting plus additional clitoral stimulation. Only 10 percent of intercourse experiences extend over 10 minutes. Typically, lovemaking including pleasuring, intercourse, and afterplay extends from 20 to 45 minutes. Intercourse is only 2-7 minutes of the lovemaking experience. A man who sets out to achieve better control solely for the woman's sake is missing the point and setting unrealistic performance demands on both he and she.

WHAT IS EJACULATORY CONTROL?

The motivation for developing ejaculatory control is realizing there is more to sexuality than intercourse and orgasm. Orgasm is important, but why focus on it to the exclusion of sensual and erotic experiences? Men are not aware of the pleasure available to them through nongenital touching, how turned on they can become through slow, tender, sensuous stimulation, and the variety of erotic scenarios and techniques they can experiment with. He can enjoy her responsivity and arousal. Not only can prolonged pleasuring and intercourse be exciting, but when he does ejaculate, orgasm is more satisfying because of the slow, tantalizing buildup.

In developing ejaculatory control, it would be best to keep our sights fixed on a happy medium rather than pursuing perfectionistic goals. There is a tendency for attitudes about ejaculation to go to extremes. In the past it was acceptable for a man to ejaculate soon after intromission. Today, any sexual encounter that does not last at least thirty minutes and result in multiple orgasms for the woman is considered a failure by the "sexually sophisticated." This performance-oriented approach sets the couple up for sexual dysfunction. The healthy association is between "sex and pleasure," not "sex and performance." When sex is viewed as a performance, you are halfway to developing a sexual dysfunction.

What exactly constitutes early ejaculation? How soon is too soon? Obviously, there are degrees of rapid ejaculation and degrees of ejaculatory control. The man is clearly an early ejaculator if he ejaculates before intromission or within 30 seconds. Beyond this, it is difficult to assign a definite time limit. The average length of intercourse is two to seven minutes. Is ejaculation after one minute too rapid? Masters and Johnson attempted to define early ejaculation in terms of percentages rather than time. Their criterion was if the woman is regularly orgasmic during intercourse, early ejaculation occurs if the man ejaculates before the woman's orgasm more than 50 percent of the time.

This definition is too performance-oriented and arbitrary. It fails to take into account individual differences in female sexual response.

The approach to defining early ejaculation is on the wrong track. The emphasis should not be on how soon is too soon, but on helping both the man and woman gain greater satisfaction from the lovemaking process, including intercourse. If the couple are making good use of nongenital and genital pleasuring and the male's ejaculation is earlier than desired and interferes with pleasure, then increasing ejaculatory control is worthwhile. Instead of viewing early ejaculation as a major dysfunction that makes the man inadequate or causes the woman to feel sexually ignored, think of ejaculatory control as a skill the couple—not just the man—develop to enhance mutual satisfaction.

LEARNING EJACULATORY CONTROL
The point is if you ejaculate more rapidly than you or your partner would like, you are experiencing a very common problem, and will find it worthwhile to improve ejaculatory control. In fact, most men would feel more comfortable with intercourse if they were more aware and open to slower, varied sensual and erotic techniques. The most reasonable way to look at ejaculatory control is as a learned skill that both the man and woman can be actively involved in acquiring to enhance the sexual enjoyment of both.

Ejaculatory control consists of two steps. The first is to be aware of the sensations just before the point of ejaculatory inevitability. Male arousal is a voluntary response up to this point, but after it orgasm becomes involuntary. He will ejaculate no matter what. When you reach the point of ejaculatory inevitability, even if your mother-in-law were to walk into the bedroom, you will ejaculate. Men who tune in to their sensations at the point of inevitability report a feeling of intense arousal, a sense of the penis being "full," and a powerful urge to let go and ejaculate. The point of ejaculatory inevitability occurs one to three seconds before the onset of ejaculation. The point of inevitability is the beginning of the orgasmic response.

Once the man is aware of the point of ejaculatory inevitability, the second step is to prolong the sensations of high arousal with-

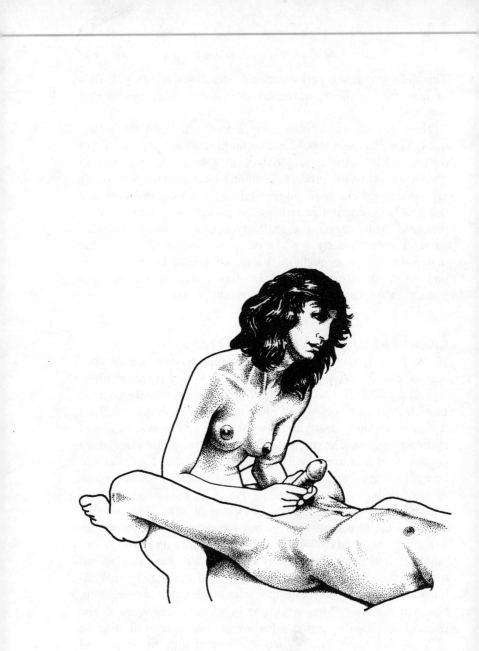

An exercise in ejaculatory control where the stop-start technique is utilized.

out moving to the point of inevitability. This strategy is the opposite of the "common sense" approach of tuning out sexual arousal by using distracting thoughts, biting the corner of the pillow, or reducing erotic stimulation. Tune in to arousal and penile sensations and learn to be comfortable with them.

Men who have a long-standing habit of early ejaculation engage in a program of exercises designed to increase their ability to control the intensity of stimulation. These exercises center around the "stop-start" technique, a method of controlling the level of sexual excitement by stopping stimulation and movement until the urge to ejaculate decreases. Although it is possible for him to use this technique by himself, more effective and lasting results will be obtained if the woman is involved and the couple employs a program of progressive exercises. Originally, a technique called the "squeeze" was utilized, but it has fallen into disfavor because people found it too mechanical. The stop-start technique is straightforward, although it requires practice and feedback to master. Couples find sex therapy is superior to self-help approaches because the structure of therapy and consultation with a professional facilitates motivation and focus as well as helps in dealing with inevitable frustrations and setbacks.

EJACULATORY CONTROL EXERCISES

During the first exercise, the couple assume a comfortable pleasuring position. The most commonly used position is he lies on his back with his legs outstretched while she sits or kneels by him so she has full access to his genitals. She utilizes manual stimulation until he feels aroused and has a firm erection. At this point she stops stimulation, causing the excitement to decrease. After 10 seconds, she resumes stimulation until he reports feeling aroused, and again stops stimulation. She is applying the stop-start before the point of ejaculatory inevitability to get them comfortable with the technique.

The next step is the man employs a signal during manual stimulation to tell her the point of inevitability is approaching. This signal can be verbal such as "Now" or "Stop," or he may motion with his hand. He signals as soon as he feels the sensations of approaching ejaculation, and she immediately ceases stimulation. The man should not try to fight his urge to ejaculate or detach from feelings of arousal. He accepts and enjoys the sensations and relies on her to help him control his ejaculatory reflex by stopping stimulation. Cessation of stimulation decreases his urge to ejaculate. They continue to use arousal and stop procedures for seven to ten minutes, even if they have to stop and start ten times. When the man ejaculates, even if it is earlier than he wants, he need not be upset, enjoy the orgasm.

This attitude remains true for subsequent exercises. If you make what you consider a "mistake" and ejaculate, don't feel you failed or did something wrong, enjoy your orgasm. The experience can be instructive as well as pleasurable, since it helps you learn to discriminate the point of ejaculatory inevitability. There is nothing magic in the stop-start technique; it is a learning process that focuses on your pattern of arousal and breaks the connection between sexual excitement and anxiety. You want to maintain high arousal and combine it with a sense of awareness and comfort.

After the couple has practiced the stop-start technique and he's ejaculated, switch roles so the man is the sexual giver. She guides him in using whatever stimulation she finds particularly arousing and satisfying. This reinforces a number of crucial concepts, including sex does not end with the man's orgasm. Partners can take turns giving and receiving sexual pleasure. Nonintercourse sex can be arousing and satisfying.

When the couple has done this enough times (usually two to four experiences) to feel comfortable, they move on to the next step. This time, the woman assumes the female on top position, with her buttocks resting on his thighs. She stimulates him, but instead of just using her hands, she rubs his penis against her vulva (although she doesn't insert the penis). Use a lotion to lubricate the penis, such as aloe vera, baby oil, Astroglide, or K-Y Jelly. Sensations are similar to those of intercourse. As soon as he feels the point of ejaculatory inevitability approaching, he immediately signals, and she stops stimulation. The couple can experiment with various kinds of stimulation until they feel comfortable and confident with their ability to prolong erotic stimulation. She might try rubbing the penis against her breasts or using fellatio.

The next exercise involves integrating ejaculatory control during intercourse. From the female on top position, she initiates and guides intromission in a slow, comfortable manner. After intromission, he lies quietly and focuses on the sensations of vaginal containment. This is called the "quiet vagina" technique. He enjoys the sensations of intravaginal containment with no performance pressure. She begins slow, rhythmic, non-demand thrusting. As soon as he feels the point of ejaculatory inevitability approaching, he signals, and she stops movement. It is possible to prolong intercourse for four to seven minutes. As comfort and control are achieved, the couple begin experimenting with prolonged coital thrusting with the man controlling thrusting and slowing stimulation rather than stopping.

Learning ejaculatory control is a gradual process. Ejaculatory control is most difficult with short, rapid thrusting in the male on top position. Couples establish ejaculatory control with other intercourse positions and use longer, slower stroking or circular thrusting before moving to man-on-top intercourse. It is a good idea to occasionally use the stop-start technique for at least six months, even after the initial problem has been overcome. This allows you to gain greater comfort and skill at prolonging and enjoying intercourse.

Alex

Early ejaculation is one of the easier sexual dysfunctions to change. The stop-start technique is, for most men, a simple and effective method for gaining ejaculatory control. Men who have been early ejaculators all their lives are surprised and pleased to discover they can overcome the problem.

Alex, a thirty-nine-year-old man in his second marriage, had a self-defeating attitude when he entered couples sex therapy. His first wife had not complained about rapid ejaculation, so he ignored the problem. Initially, his second wife said nothing, but her resentment built. It came out six months after they were married in a blistering attack in which she claimed Alex was selfish, inconsiderate, and cared nothing for her as a person or her sexual feelings. Alex was stunned. Her accusations were upsetting and depressing. He felt emotionally wounded and angry at having these demands thrown at him. Most of all, he felt hopeless; he realized he had been an early ejaculator all his life and feared it was too late to change.

When his wife suggested he consult a therapist, Alex refused, saying he was not the kind of person who went to therapy. Soon afterward, however, they learned about couples sex therapy which Alex felt would be less objectionable. As treatment progressed, it became clear part of Alex's anxiety was caused by his reluctance to tell a male therapist he needed help. Once he accepted the idea that developing ejaculatory control was like learning any other skill and he and his wife would approach the problem as an intimate team, he became involved and cooperative.

Alex found learning ejaculatory control enjoyable as well as beneficial. The exercises were effective, and Alex was amazed to discover a problem which had been with him for so long could be successfully addressed. Alex wanted things to progress more rapidly than they did. This is a common male complaint. Men want immediate results instead of enjoying the gradual process of nondemand pleasuring, communicating with the partner, and gaining comfort and confidence with a variety of sexual scenarios and techniques.

Alex offers a good example of the value of consulting a therapist rather than trying to change on your own. A competent professional can provide guidance, keep the process on track, monitor problems that arise, and support the couple in dealing with anxiety or discouragement. The therapist encourages the couple to maintain a regular rhythm of touching and intercourse. If you only have intercourse once a week, it is difficult to develop ejaculatory control. The couple discusses ways to maintain a pleasurable and satisfying sexual relationship, so they are not vulnerable to relapse.

USE OF MEDICATION FOR EJACULATORY CONTROL

As part of a larger trend to "medicalize" male sexuality, there has been an astonishing increase in the use of low doses of antidepressant medication (Anafranil, Prozac, Zoloft) to treat early ejaculation. The data is clear in two respects: 1) ejaculatory delay does occur; 2) men prefer to take medication as opposed to engaging in sex therapy. What is less clear is the effect on the couple and how to maintain ejaculatory control. Many women object to the use of a pill instead of the man talking to and working with her. Just as importantly, will ejaculatory control continue after he stops taking medication? For most couples, unless they slow down the sexual process, communicate feelings and desires, value sensuality and pleasuring, change intercourse positions and modes of intercourse thrusting, ejaculatory control does not continue after the man stops medication.

For males with severe ejaculatory problems or couples frustrated or disappointed with the ejaculatory control process, medication is a helpful intervention. The trap is being totally dependent on the pill, rather than seeing it as an additional resource to learn ejaculatory control. If they utilize ejaculatory control exercises while he's taking medication, the benefits will maintain after he stops medication. We are wary of using medical or medication interventions as a substitute for psychological and relationship changes. The man has to be willing to deal with sexual feelings and attitudes, not ignore or avoid them. Sexuality is a couple process of giving and receiving pleasure-oriented touching. The woman is aware and involved, your intimate friend. Don't use medication as a way to shut her out.

MALES WITHOUT PARTNERS

So far, we have been speaking exclusively about men who have wives or partners willing to work with them. What about the single man who does not have a regular partner?

Although it will take longer to learn ejaculatory control, it is possible to make progress on his own. He can use the stop-start technique while masturbating, stimulating himself to the point of ejaculatory inevitability and then stopping. He does this for five to ten minutes before ejaculating. This is effective in breaking the connection between excitement and anxiety. However, the single man should not be surprised or disappointed if the control he has achieved in masturbation does not have an immediate effect during partner sex. There are a multitude of emotional and interpersonal factors which complicates the task of putting his newly learned skill into practice. However, if he is open with the partner and there is an ongoing, cooperative relationship, ejaculatory control will improve with time.

The majority of men ejaculate rapidly in initial intercourse experiences with a new partner. A man (or the woman involved) should not take it as a sign he is selfish, doesn't care for her, or is a sexual failure. His control will improve if he and his partner communicate, slow down, enjoy the pleasuring process, focus on enhancing erotic sensations, and increase involvement and awareness during intercourse. He can spend more time on tender, slow pleasuring. If he continues to ejaculate rapidly, he should not disparage himself, but enjoy the orgasmic experience. Sex does not have to end with ejaculation. He can continue to stimulate his partner and bring her to orgasm manually or by rubbing stimulation. Orgasm through nonintercourse sex can be just as enjoyable as one that occurs during intercourse. Many couples utilize manual or oral stimulation of the woman to orgasm before proceeding to intercourse. In fact, the most typical pattern for American couples is for the woman to be orgasmic during pleasuring and then proceed to intercourse where he's orgasmic. There is no reason for the man to feel he is less masculine because he has given pleasure with his mouth, body, or fingers.

CLOSING THOUGHTS

Developing ejaculatory control is like learning any new skill. First you have to decide you want to learn and keep your motivation high enough to go through the steps to achieve it. Realize it takes time, practice and feedback. Don't become angry or discouraged if you do not experience immediate improvement. Ejaculatory control is best learned as a couple, so you need to work together, support each other, communicate clearly, and avoid falling into the traps of guilt or blaming. In mastering ejaculatory control you are not only learning a specific skill, you are learning to communicate intimately and enhance your sexual repertoire. Use increased ejaculatory ability to make sex more pleasurable for you as an individual and as a couple.

15
AROUSAL AND ERECTION

Difficulty achieving or maintaining an erection is very distressing. The term traditionally used indicates how devastating the condition is felt to be: *impotence*—without potency, without strength. A man might be able to operate a jackhammer or manage an office with 100 employees, but if his penis does not become stiff when he wants it to, he is considered a flawed person. Worse yet, he considers himself a failure as a man. He denigrates himself, ignoring his attributes and accomplishments, convinced that anyone suffering from erectile dysfunction cannot be a successful man. The term *erectile dysfunction* is preferable because it's more descriptive without being emotion-laden and pejorative. It's the penis, not his whole self, that is malfunctioning. A male depends too much on his penis for his self-esteem.

There is no reason erectile dysfunction should strike such terror in the male heart. Not that there is an easy or miracle cure for erectile problems—there isn't. However, the majority of men can and do learn to regain comfort and confidence with erections. Erectile dysfunction is not the sexual death sentence it is portrayed to be. In fact, erectile problems are extremely common. By age forty, 90 percent of men have experienced at least one occasion when they could not get or maintain an erection sufficient for intercourse. For the majority of men, it is a temporary state, a rare and atypical occurrence. For one-third, the erection problems last longer, a few weeks or months, but eventually sexual functioning returns. Approximately 10 to 15 percent of men suffer with intermittent or chronic erectile dysfunction. This increases with age, so by age 50 about one in three males have mild to severe erectile dysfunction.[13] In the majority of cases, the cause is psychological or relational rather than medical. The reason the condition becomes chronic is that, like any psychological problem, it becomes self-perpetuating. Erectile dysfunction becomes more severe with time because it feeds on the performance anxiety it produces.

The performance anxiety responsible for perpetuating erectile problems, however irrational, is nevertheless extremely real. It does little good to tell a man it's all in his head (this is too simplistic and a put-down). He needs help in regaining sexual comfort and confidence. The first thing is to be aware of information about arousal and erections and formulate positive, realistic expectations.

FACTS ABOUT ERECTILE FUNCTION AND DYSFUNCTION

When we speak of erectile problems, we mean the inability to obtain or maintain an erection sufficient for intercourse. The problem is categorized as either primary or secondary—the latter by far the more common. A male with secondary erectile dysfunction has had at least one successful intercourse. Most men have had intercourse a great many times, but then experience intermittent episodes in which they cannot obtain an erection or, more commonly, achieve an erection and then lose it, typically just prior to intromission. The male with primary erectile dysfunction has never had successful intercourse—a rarer condition, but more frequent than commonly believed. He is able to masturbate to orgasm, and is often able to achieve erections and orgasm through manual or oral stimulation. He feels humiliated and embarrassed and sees erectile dysfunction as evidence of inadequacy as a person. He needs to realize there is more to him and his sexuality than the state of his penis.

Erection is not the automatic result of an erotic stimulus. Rather, a man becomes aroused when he is feeling comfortable with himself and his partner and is open to pleasure. Being receptive to touch sets the stage for eroticism, arousal and erection. Erection is not a voluntary occurrence. A man cannot will an erection or force himself to obtain one. In fact, the more he obsesses about getting an erection and focuses on the state of his penis, the less likely he is to feel aroused. Erection is the end result of a chain of psychological and physiological events. If there are links in the chain that are missing, erection will be blocked. Erection is a natural physiological response that can be subverted by a number of factors, including anticipatory anxiety, performance anxiety, anger, depression, fatigue, alcohol, medication side effects, and distraction.

When an erection fails to occur, the problem usually lies at the very beginning of the sexual response cycle. The man might be tired, depressed, frustrated, preoccupied, or just not interested in sex at the moment. By trying to have intercourse anyway— to oblige his partner or because it is expected—he is going against his feelings and desires. He's not receptive to erotic stimuli. Inability to have or maintain an erection under circumstances where he is anxious or distracted is natural and understandable.

A different situation occurs when a man has had too much to drink—the most common cause of situational erectile dysfunction. Although an inebriated man may feel amorous and uninhibited, physiologically his sexual functioning is impaired. Men who experience erectile dysfunction after drinking become anxious about their ability to perform. Anxiety may lead to inability to get or maintain erections on later occasions, when he is sober. The cycle of anticipatory anxiety, performance pressure and sexual avoidance has been activated.

Benjamin

This is the pattern a client of Barry's, Benjamin, a successful forty-six-year-old salesman for a boat-building concern, was stuck in. Benjamin was a heavy drinker, and during a period in his life when there was increased job pressure, combined with concern about his teenage son, he developed an alcohol abuse pattern. Benjamin became quite drunk at a party. When they arrived home, he tried to have sex but was unable to keep an erection. His wife was supportive and understood it was because of the alcohol, but the episode worried and depressed Benjamin. When he attempted intercourse the next day, he initially achieved an erection but was unable to maintain it. This pattern worsened. Sometimes he maintained an erection, but most of the time he didn't. As soon as he became erect, he immediately attempted intromission because he feared he'd lose it. Eventually, he stopped attempting sex. The negative anticipation, tension filled sexual performance and sexual avoidance pattern controlled their sexual relationship.

Benjamin's initial erectile problem resulted from a combination of alcohol with family and business pressures, but he was unable to accept this perspective. The drinking became out of control and Benjamin was forced to admit he was an alcoholic. With the aid of Alcoholics Anonymous, he abstained from drinking, but the erection problem remained. It is not unusual, even when the initial problem is resolved, that the erectile problem continues because of the anticipatory and performance anxiety cycle.

At the point they entered sex therapy, Benjamin was quite negative. He'd given up hope of ever regaining erectile functioning. Eventually, however, he began to understand the connection between anxiety and erection. He and his wife began nongenital and genital pleasuring exercises with the focus on comfort, pleasure and eroticism. There was a temporary prohibition on intercourse which reduced performance anxiety. A key experience was learning his erection could wax and wane and wax again. He no longer panicked nor felt compelled to jump on his first erection. In a matter of three months, Benjamin was getting erections and having intercourse 85 percent of the time. Other times they would enjoy sensual pleasuring or non-intercourse sex to orgasm. As his wife said, they developed a broader, more flexible sexual repertoire. Sex was more fun and varied, not as predictable.

AUTOMATIC ERECTIONS

The majority of men respond to an erectile problem just as Benjamin did. They ignore the importance of the initial, less obvious links in the chain of sexual arousal—namely, feelings of comfort and receptivity. They make the erroneous assumption that erection should follow automatically whenever the opportunity for sex presents itself. They believe the myth of the male machine that a "real man" can have sex anytime, anyplace, with any woman. The most sensible response a man can have to erectile problems is to interpret it as a sign he does not really want to have sex at the moment—just as he would interpret the lack of an appetite as a sign he should not order a three course meal. He might tell his partner, "I'm not in the mood for intercourse right now." Or he could request she give him a massage—something to relax him and facilitate receptivity and responsivity. He might offer to "give to her" manually or orally.

But men with erectile problems do not respond in this way. The most common reaction is panic and desperation. Rather than relaxing and requesting she use stimulation that is pleasurable and arousing, he avoids sharing his concerns or involving her. He may try to force arousal, pretending a level of passion he does not feel. He attempts to achieve intromission with a fading erection. The sexual interaction ends on a note of frustration for both partners, with misunderstanding and resentment on each side. The man feels he is a failure and the woman alternates between blaming herself and blaming him. The next time he feels even more pressure to "redeem his manhood" with an "A" level sexual performance. He is controlled by anticipatory and performance anxiety. The vicious cycle of negative anticipation, failed performance, and sexual avoidance is reinforced. What started as a normal occurrence is on its way to becoming a tragedy.

EFFECT ON THE RELATIONSHIP

In addition to the havoc it wreaks on the man's self-esteem, an erection problem is detrimental to his relationship. Erectile problems are usually traced to performance anxiety, distraction, misunderstanding, and lack of communication. It is very difficult to explain to himself or his partner what is happening. Since he believes it is a sign of masculinity to perform flawlessly in every sexual encounter, he is filled with an overwhelming desire to cover up his failure or find an excuse for it. Faced with this need to find a scapegoat, he may try to pin the blame on his partner, letting her believe erectile problems stem from the fact he finds her unattractive or she turns him off. She may retaliate by ridiculing him for his failure to perform. In a very short time the relationship becomes tense and hostile. This is opposite of what he needs. Erection problems are best conceptualized and treated as a couple issue. He needs to think of her as his intimate friend.

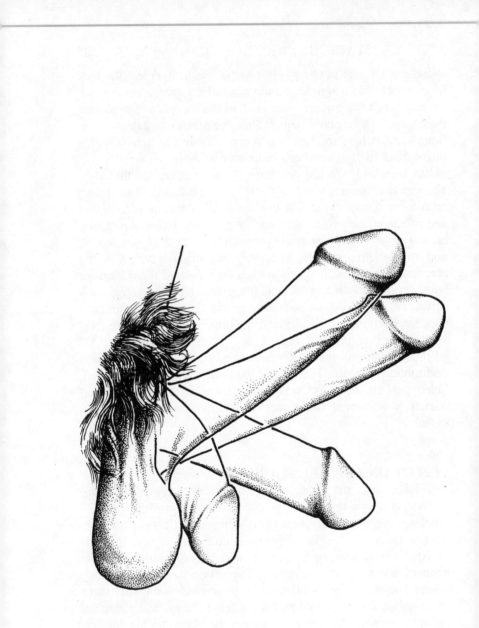

The four states of arousal. Erection is triggered by nerve centers in the lower spinal column signaling blood to enter the penis through arteries running through the erectile tissue.

Working together as an intimate team they can develop a comfortable, pleasurable, erotic, and functional couple sexual style.

Another counterproductive response is to make a play for her sympathy. The excuses he makes to explain his erectile dysfunction are accurate—overwork, tiredness, pressure, anxiety, distraction—only the attitude is wrong. If the woman responds as he wants her to, by showing pity and acting maternal, the situation becomes worse. Her sympathy, in effect, becomes a crutch, which makes it harder for him to feel sexual. What he needs is not pity, sympathy or condescension, but a partner who is willing to see the erectile dysfunction as a mutual problem and work with him in regaining sexual comfort and confidence. Her sexual pleasure and arousal is a friend to their sexual relationship—her arousal facilitates his arousal.

While on the subject of the woman's role, let us consider a thesis that has gained a following in recent years—namely, erectile dysfunction is increasing as a result of the intimidating effect of the women's movement. The argument is that as women become more sexually assertive, more unwilling to serve as a passive "vessel" for male gratification, the pressure on men to perform becomes so great they feel overwhelmed, and the result is erectile failure. It is true there has been an increase in the number of males experiencing erectile problems. Partly this is a reflection of the greater freedom to discuss sexual problems and the fact there are now treatment programs for sexual dysfunction, which was not true a generation ago. But this does not address the question of whether the assertive attitudes and sexual awareness espoused by the women's movement have a negative effect on male sexuality.

The best aphrodisiac is an active, involved partner. The woman who is aware of her sexuality, makes clear and direct sexual requests, and is sexually responsive, increases male arousal. The woman's capacity for sexual pleasure is at least as great as the man's. There is no possible justification for denying women the opportunity to enjoy their sexuality. Some men, especially those who identify strongly with traditional ideas of male dominance, are threatened by this model of male-female sexual equity. But this calls for a change in male attitudes not a suppression of female sexual response.

Males are unaware that on some occasions women are more

sexually responsive and orgasmic than men. The double standard has led them to believe it is always the man who is the sexual aggressor and enjoys sex more. When a woman is assertive, highly responsive, and multiorgasmic, traditionalist men feel threatened. This results in losing erectile confidence. Other men see sexual sharing as positive. It means their partner is motivated to be responsive, take initiatives, and to be a sexually creative intimate friend. These men find a woman's receptivity and responsivity is a stimulant. In a healthy sexual relationship both the man and woman are free to initiate and both can say no or propose an alternative. The man has a right to say no, request time to play, or suggest erotic scenarios and techniques. The woman's initiation is a request for sexual pleasure, not a demand for sexual performance. This attitude is the logical and productive one. If more men adopted it, there would be little cause for concern about the effects of the women's movement on erectile functioning.

ASSESSING ERECTION PROBLEMS

The most urgent question the man with an erection problem has is what to do about it. The first step is to not panic or overreact. Erectile response is multicausal and multidimensional and so is erectile dysfunction. Perhaps the most important assessment issue is, can the man obtain an erection by other means? For example, the male who is able to get firm erections with masturbation, manual stimulation, or oral sex can be reasonably confident the problem is caused primarily by psychological, relationship, or situational factors. For men who report few or no erections or lack of sexual desire, it is worthwhile to consult your general physician before or concurrent with consulting a sex therapist.

Physiologically, three systems need to be functional for erections to occur—hormonal, vascular, and neurological. Any factor which has a negative impact on your general health can affect sexuality. The most common physical cause of erectile problems is side effects of medication, especially implicated are medications for hypertension. Other common causes are poorly controlled diabetes, vascular disorders, alcohol or drug abuse, smoking, endocrine disorders which affect testosterone, and neurological disorders. The internist might suggest a consultation with an urologist, the physician closest to the female equivalent of a gynecologist. Make sure the urologist is interested in doing a comprehensive evaluation rather than promoting penile injections, external pump devices, oral medication or prosthesis surgery.

Contrary to the widespread belief, even among physicians, that a medical problem will always result in a sexual dysfunction, most males with medical problems do not develop erectile dysfunction. For example, men who are diabetic do not necessarily develop sexual problems. Barry is an adult onset diabetic who maintains a diet and exercise program. His diabetes is under good control and has not impacted sexual functioning. Men with chronic medical conditions need to be aware of the potential problems and be an active patient in enhancing physical well-being and preventing sexual dysfunction.

MEDICAL INTERVENTIONS

When there are significant physiological factors which impair erectile function, the urologist or sexual medicine specialist will review the medical alternatives for dealing with erectile dysfunction. Ideally, this would be discussed with your spouse or partner. Choose a treatment which can be comfortably integrated into your sexual relationship. As a caveat, what we write now will change dramatically in the next few years. Researchers are trying to develop user-friendly medical interventions.

The most invasive treatment is a surgical procedure—a penile prothesis. This is a major surgery involving general anesthesia and a hospital stay of several days. The prothesis guarantees an erection suitable for intercourse so anxiety about failed intercourse is eliminated. There are two types of prostheses—an inflatable mechanism or semirigid rods. Each type has a drawback—men with the rods feel uncomfortable and self-conscious about always having a semi-erection. Because it's more mechanically complicated, men fear the pump malfunctioning or wearing out so another surgery would be necessary. The biggest drawback is prosthesis surgery is not reversible, since vascular and neurological structures are disrupted by the surgery. The penile prosthesis was an important breakthrough in the treatment of organic erectile dysfunction, but because of its irreversibility it needs to be considered very carefully. Many men are attracted to it as a return to automatic erections and a magical cure for all sexual problems. However, the penile prothesis does not affect desire or orgasm, and most important, it doesn't guarantee emotional satisfaction for the man or woman.

A second alternative is an injection of a vasodilator into the penis before intercourse. This results in a firm erection which can last from 45 minutes to 4 hours. Once he's used the injection, the woman's penile stimulation enhances the erection. It can be utilized 2-3 times a week. Although many men adapt well to self-injections, a substantial number drop out of treatment in less than a year. Reasons include lack of spontaneity, dislike over doing injections, and partner resistance. Some men report increased discomfort or pain after months of injections. The most common reason for discontinuing is the couple do not successfully integrate injections into their lovemaking style. Paradoxically, this is given as an advantage, especially for single men. They can keep the technique secret from the partner. Men who enjoy the injection technique report freedom from fear of failure. The injection allows them to bypass performance anxiety. Another advantage is after they ejaculate they can continue intercourse if desired by the partner.

The external vacuum pump is the least expensive medical alternative, with no worries about long-term side effects. The man uses the pump (which must be prescribed by a physician) to create an erection and then places a band (ring) around the base of the penis to retain vasocongestion and penile firmness. The erection lasts approximately half an hour. The woman can, and is encouraged, to stimulate his penis once he's erect. The major plus of the external pump is it's reasonably easy to use, will lead to successful intercourse aproximately 75 percent of the time, and freedom from side effects. The disadvantage is the planned, mechanical nature of the mechanism. Some men (and women) do not enjoy the sensations of the penis. If the ring is too tight, it is difficult to ejaculate. There is a fear of losing firmness if pleasuring or intercourse is extended.

These medical interventions are functional, but not ''user friendly.'' The intervention receiving a good deal of experimental attention is an oral medication which could be used an hour before having sex. This medication would have an activating vasodilating effect. With sexual pleasuring and direct penile stimulation it results in naturally occurring erections. The hope is oral medication would not have side effects. Separating the medical intervention from lovemaking is a positive so the man is more likely to continue with the medication.

Even when the cause of an erection problem is primarily vascular or neurological, it is still possible to enjoy other erotic techniques and have an orgasm without a firm erection. Many couples choose to enter sex therapy and adapt their sexual style so it is less dependent on intercourse.

The man and his partner need to understand the medical, psychological, and relational aspects of the erection problem. They can thoughtfully discuss whether they would benefit from sex therapy, marital therapy, a medical intervention, or a combination of approaches.

SEX THERAPY INTERVENTIONS

When a man tries to make his penis erect by force of will, the result is a strained and anxious focusing on the penis. Because it is not humanly possible to concentrate on two things at the same time, feelings of pleasure and eroticism diminish. He becomes detached from the erotic flow, an anxious spectator intent only upon detecting signs of arousal, yet oblivious to the erotic stimuli that cause it. Sex is not a spectator sport; you have to be an involved partner in giving and receiving pleasure and erotic stimulation. The following guidelines are used by men in sex therapy to increase understanding, awareness, and comfort with a range of sexual scenarios and techniques.

AROUSAL AND ERECTION GUIDELINES

1. By age forty, 90 percent of males experience at least one erectile failure; this is a normal occurrence, not a sign of erectile dysfunction.
2. The majority of erectile problems are caused by psychological or relationship factors, not medical or physiolog-

ical malfunctions. To evaluate medical factors consult an urologist with training in erectile function and dysfunction.

3. Erectile problems can be caused by a wide variety of factors including alcohol, anxiety, depression, distraction, anger, side effects of medication, frustration, fatigue, not feeling sexual at that time or with that partner.

4. The key is to view the erectile difficulty as a situational problem, not overreact and label yourself "impotent" or put yourself down as a "failure."

5. Don't believe the myth of the "male machine," ready to have an erection and intercourse at any time, with any woman, in any situation. You and your penis are human. You are not a performance machine.

6. A pervasive myth is if a man loses his initial erection, it means he's sexually turned off. It is a natural physiological process for erections to wax and wane during prolonged pleasuring.

7. In a typical forty-five-minute pleasuring session, the male's erection will wax and wane two to five times. Subsequent erections, intercourse, and orgasm are quite satisfying.

8. You don't need an erect penis to satisfy a woman. Orgasm can be achieved through manual, oral, or rubbing stimulation. If you have problems getting or maintaining an erection, don't stop the sexual interaction. Many women find it arousing to have the partner's fingers, tongue, or penis (erect or flaccid) used for stimulation.

9. Involve yourself actively in giving and receiving pleasurable touching. Erection is a natural result of pleasure, eroticism, and arousal.

10. You cannot will or force an erection. Avoid being a passive "spectator" who observes the state of his penis. Sex is not a spectator sport, it requires active involvement.

11. Allow the woman to initiate intercourse and guide your penis into her vagina. This reduces performance pressure and, since the woman is the expert on her vagina, is the most practical procedure.

12. Feel comfortable saying, "I want sex and pleasuring to be nondemanding. When I feel pressure to perform, I get

uptight and sex is not good. Let's make sexuality enjoyable by taking it at a comfortable pace and being an intimate team.''

13. Erectile problems do not affect the ability to ejaculate (men can ejaculate with a flaccid penis). The man can relearn to ejaculate to the cue of an erect penis.

14. One way to regain comfort and confidence is through masturbation. During masturbation you can practice gaining and losing erections, relearn ejaculating with an erect penis, and focus on fantasies and stimulation which will transfer to partner sex.

15. Don't try to use your morning erection for intercourse. This erection is associated with REM sleep or results from being close to your partner. Men try vainly to have intercourse with their morning erections before they lose them. Remember: arousal and erection are regainable. Morning is a good time to be sexual.

16. Make clear, direct, assertive requests (not demands) for the sexual stimulation you find most erotic and arousing. Verbally and nonverbally guide your partner in how to pleasure and arouse you.

17. Stimulating a flaccid penis is counterproductive, the man becomes obsessed with the state of his penis. Instead, engage in sensuous, nondemand stimulation. Enjoy giving and receiving stimulation rather than trying to "will an erection."

18. Attitudes and self-thoughts influence arousal. The key is "sex and pleasure" not "sex and performance."

19. Feelings about a sexual experience are best measured by pleasure and satisfaction, not whether you got an erection, how hard it was, or whether your partner was orgasmic. Some sexual experiences will be great for both of you, some will be better for one than the other, some will be mediocre, and others will be poor or downright failures. Do not put your sexual self-esteem on the line at each sexual experience.

20. When sleeping, you get an erection every ninety minutes—three to five erections a night. Sex is a natural physiological function. Don't block it by anticipatory anxiety, performance anxiety, distraction, or putting yourself

down. Give yourself (and your partner) permission to enjoy the pleasure of sexuality.

ERECTILE EXERCISES

A couple can deal with an erectile problem through engaging in exercises to increase sexual awareness. We strongly suggest doing these with the guidance and support of a sex therapist. The chief causes of erection problems are performance anxiety and distraction. The remedy is to regain sexual comfort and confidence.

Begin by having a quiet, intimate talk over a drink (limit it to one glass, alcohol is a central nervous system depressant) or coffee, followed by a relaxing, sensuous shower. Lather each other all over, including the genitals, then dry your partner. Be sure you have time and privacy to enjoy the experience. Go into the bedroom and get into a comfortable position for pleasuring. The woman starts as giver, with the man as recipient. She begins by stroking his chest or thighs; gradually moving toward his genitals. The man is open to feelings of pleasure rather than worrying whether he is getting erect. If the man is receptive and the woman continues to pleasure him in a sensuous, nondemand way, an erection will occur. At this point, pleasuring ceases and the couple lie comfortably together until the erection subsides.

Be aware of your feelings at this moment. How do you feel as the penis returns to a flaccid state—anxious, worried, tense, angry, relieved? Gaining confidence an erection will return after it has subsided is vital. A psychological trap for a man is as soon as he gets erect, he feels pressure to use it because of fear he'll lose it. This is especially true with his morning erection. When the erection dissipates before intercourse, as it usually does, he becomes frustrated and depressed—two emotions that block arousal.

After a minute, the couple resume pleasuring. Be open and receptive, accept and enjoy feelings of pleasure. Let yourself respond to each touch. Allow your body to drink in each feeling. When an erection occurs, again lie quietly together until it subsides. In understanding the natural physiological process of waxing and waning of erections, the man has taken a giant step forward. Young men are used to "automatic erections" and always having intercourse on their first erection. You can enjoy sex more and be a better lover by engaging in sensuous, pleasure-oriented touching, view sexuality as a giving, intimate experience rather than an automatic response. Pleasure, arousal, and erection is a process. Sex is not a narrow window of opportunity where you either have intercourse on the first erection or you fail.

Reverse positions, letting the man take the role of giver and enjoy giving pleasure. An erection may occur naturally. If so, enjoy the sensations and continue pleasuring her.

Continue until both of you are comfortable with the man gaining and losing an erection. The point is to help him focus on sensual and erotic sensations. He becomes comfortable with the natural process of erections without being anxious about performance. It is normal for a man's penis to become alternately hard and soft during an extended pleasuring session. During a forty-five minute pleasuring experience, the male's erection will wax and wane an average of two to five times. The ensuing orgasm is more pleasurable after this tantalizing buildup. The erection partially or entirely disappearing need not be a cause for anxiety or alarm. Becoming anxious or distracted, or working hard to bring it back, is self-defeating.

For the second exercise, use the female on top intercourse position. The prohibition on intercourse remains. This exercise will accustom both partners to having the penis close to and in contact with the vulva. To increase comfort, place a pillow under her thighs and one under his head. She begins caressing and stimulating and he's free to request specific stimulation and guide her in touching which increases erotic sensations. If the man becomes anxious or worried, rather than giving in to distracting thoughts, he tells her what he's feeling. Together, they become reinvolved in the sexual interaction. He could do this by pleasuring her or making a clear, direct request for specific stimulation such as "rub the underside of my penis with just your fingertips."

When he gets an erection, instead of letting it subside, she takes the penis and rubs it around her vulva. She uses the glans of the penis to stimulate her mons, labia, and clitoris, but does not insert it into the vagina. If he begins to lose the erection or shows signs of becoming tense, she should not stop, but return

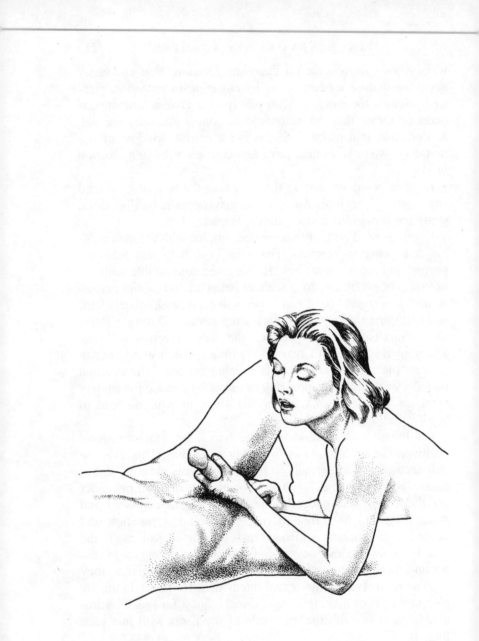

Arousal and erection are not automatic. Erection is the result of responsivity to erotic stimulation.

to fondling and caressing the penis, testicles, and inner thighs. She can use manual or oral stimulation, and he is free to stimulate her at the same time. Use of multiple stimulation, including fantasy, is key in building and maintaining sexual arousal. Remember, it is normal for the penis to become alternately hard and soft during pleasuring. The exercise ends with the couple switching positions and the man pleasuring the woman, using the kind of stimulation she enjoys most. Many men find mutual pleasuring or giving to the woman more arousing because his active involvement is the best way to counter distracting thoughts.

For the third exercise, begin with playful mutual touching. Be aware of the erotic flow—from comfort to pleasure to eroticism to high arousal. The woman can use a variety of pleasuring techniques. She decides when to move from pleasuring to intercourse. From the female-on-top position, she initiates and guides intromission. He can stimulate her or not—whichever feels best. If she notices any tension, she can resume manual or oral stimulation. Intercourse is not separate from the erotic process—it's not the pass-fail test of sex. Intercourse is best conceptualized as a special pleasuring technique; a natural extension of pleasuring, not separate from it.

Both the man and woman are aware a firm erection is not necessary for intromission. With the woman's guidance and active participation, a semi-erect penis is relatively easy to insert into the vagina. It is a good technique for the woman to initiate the moment of intercourse and guide the penis into her vagina. This takes the pressure off the man. Since she is the expert on her sexuality, it is reasonable for her to guide his penis into her.

The couple begins slow, rhythmic thrusting. There is a tendency to thrust vigorously to quickly build eroticism, but this is not necessary. Allow intercourse to be involving and rhythmic. Most men find multiple stimulation during intercourse increases arousal. Experience and accept the pleasurable, erotic sensations of intercourse. You're free to proceed to orgasm. Later, try other intercourse positions. You can experiment with "quickies," take turns guiding intromission, and vary the type and rhythm of coital thrusting.

MAINTAINING ERECTILE COMFORT AND CONFIDENCE

Erection is a natural result of effective sexual stimulation as long as nothing is inhibiting pleasure or distracting from the erotic flow. The basis of erectile response is receptivity and pleasure, performance anxiety and self-consciousness subvert erectile function. One way to block arousal is for the man to give way to anxiety and try to will an erection, becoming a spectator in the sexual interaction. It is crucial he remain active in giving and receiving pleasurable touching. In addition, there must be erotic stimulation. Men who are performance oriented rather than pleasure oriented have a great deal of trouble requesting specific erotic scenarios and techniques. Faced with erectile difficulties, they are likely to remain silent, struggling with the problem, rather than saying "Honey, I really want to make love, but I'm a little out of it right now. Could you caress my penis the way you did last Thursday?" A man can't have intercourse alone, and neither can he deal with erectile problems alone.

The key is the one-two-three combination of intimate communication, nondemand pleasuring, and erotic stimulation. Erection problems occur when there is a breakdown in communication because one partner is tired, anxious, distracted, worried, preoccupied, or distressed. The way to deal with erection problems, or any sexual dysfunction, is to reestablish intimate communication, focus on pleasuring, build eroticism, and see erection and intercourse as a natural extension of the pleasuring process.

16

OVERCOMING EJACULATORY INHIBITION

Ejaculatory inhibition—the inability to ejaculate during partner sex—has the reputation of being a rare and exotic sexual dysfunction. It is usually given short shift, often not mentioned in sexual books or discussions about sexual problems. Ejaculatory inhibition is less common than erectile dysfunction or early ejaculation. Yet, this problem confronts 5 to 15 percent of males. There are different forms of ejaculatory inhibition—from the total inability to ejaculate to the specific inability to ejaculate during intercourse. The most common type affects middle-years men, and involves intermittent problems reaching orgasm during intercourse.

The man with ejaculatory inhibition is able to be aroused, gets and maintains an erection, but has great difficulty or is unable to reach orgasm. When this occurs at rare intervals, it's frustrating, baffling, and anxiety producing, but the ability to ejaculate soon returns. Men are not perfectly functioning sexual machines, so occasional problems are best thought of as normal variability. There is no reason to worry or develop performance anxiety. However, when it continues over a period of weeks or occurs more than 25 percent of the time, the man needs to take the problem seriously and investigate ways to overcome ejaculatory inhibition.

Some men are able to reach orgasm during masturbation, but not with a partner. Most men only have this problem during intercourse, but others are unable to ejaculate during manual or oral stimulation. Most men are able to be orgasmic during self-stimulation with the partner present. Although this condition has acute psychological and, in many cases, physical effects, it has not been taken seriously by either experts or the general public. Let us examine why this is so.

CONFUSION ABOUT EJACULATORY INHIBITION

First there is the matter of terminology. Since ejaculatory inhibition has not been studied as extensively as other sexual dysfunctions, there is less consensus about its characteristics. This uncertainty is reflected in the variety of terms that have been used to describe the problem, including "ejaculatory incompetence," "retarded ejaculation," and "ejaculatory inability." "Ejaculatory inhibition" is preferable because it is the least value laden and most accurately describes the problem. The inability to ejaculate or difficulty in ejaculation stems from some type of inhibition—inability to let go, to fully enjoy sexual arousal, share intimacy and eroticism, make specific sexual requests, allow arousal to naturally culminate in orgasm. Ejaculatory inhibition is not to be confused with retrograde ejaculation, a physiological condition in which orgasm occurs, but the semen goes into the bladder rather than being ejaculated from the penis. This is a side effect of prostate surgery. Ejaculatory inhibition is also not to be confused with the naturally occurring phenomenon in men over sixty of a lessened need to ejaculate at each sexual opportunity. Ejaculatory inhibition is a problem for the male who is aroused and desires to ejaculate, but is unable to do so.

Ejaculatory inhibition has received so little attention because of two widespread and inaccurate assumptions. The first is ejaculatory inhibition is a problem only when it occurs in its most severe form, total inability to ejaculate during intercourse, thus interfering with conception. The second is because of "lasting power," he is able to satisfy his partner to an extraordinary degree. While he may miss the pleasure of orgasm, he has the consolation of knowing he is a superlative lover. We call this the "blessing in disguise" assumption.

The first assumption discounts the reality that ejaculatory inhibition is associated with a reduction in sexual pleasure and couple satisfaction. He has an erection and intercourse, but with coital thrusting over a long period of time is unable to climax. As he becomes more frustrated and focused on ejaculatory performance, his level of arousal declines, and eventually he loses his erection. "Ah ha," he says, "I have an erection problem!" He is mislabeling the dysfunction, the loss of erection is caused by ejaculatory inhibition. In other cases, the man pushes himself so hard to reach orgasm and focuses so narrowly on maintaining arousal that, while he does manage to ejaculate, neither intercourse nor ejaculation is pleasurable for him (or his partner). The result? Waning interest in sex. Because of unfamiliarity with the underlying cause, he mislabels the dysfunction as inhibited sexual desire. The common element is the erotic flow of moving from desire to pleasure to eroticism to arousal to orgasm is inhibited. As a result, the man stops anticipating sex. Rather than orgasm being the natural culmination of an erotic and arousing sexual experience, it becomes an anxiety-provoking goal he often fails to achieve. Frustration is multiplied for the man and his spouse if they desire to get pregnant.

The second assumption—the "blessing in disguise"—represents male glorification of performance over pleasure. What it overlooks is mutual pleasure is the key to sexual satisfaction. Ejaculatory inhibition greatly decreases pleasure for the man, so there is little real satisfaction for either partner. The first few times the woman might be surprised and pleased by his performance; she enjoys orgasm with intercourse. However, unless she is totally oblivious, she soon becomes aware of his lack of pleasure. If intercourse continues for half an hour and he has not ejaculated, he will experience physical discomfort as a result of continued high level of vasocongestion. This condition, commonly known as "blue balls," is not harmful, but is acutely uncomfortable. She finds prolonged intercourse physically painful because her lubrication dries up and she's not enjoying prolonged thrusting. The great majority of women who are orgasmic during intercourse will be orgasmic within 10 minutes of thrusting. After a half hour of intercourse neither the man nor the woman is turned on, and she's physically and emotionally irritated.

CAUSES OF EJACULATORY INHIBITION

Like most sexual problems, ejaculatory inhibition is multicausal. Causes usually are psychological rather than physical, involving one or more inhibitions. These include negative sexual experiences (guilt over a sexually traumatic incident or an unwanted pregnancy), fear of contracting HIV/AIDS, inadequate or inappropriate sexual learning (an idiosyncratic masturbation pattern or compulsive masturbation to a fetish stimulus), anger at the partner, lack of effective sexual stimulation, beginning intercourse before feeling subjectively aroused, shyness about requesting partner stimulation, putting the woman's sexual needs before his. Physical causes should be evaluated, particularly if the man is unable to ejaculate under any circumstances. Consult a urologist or sexual medicine specialist to determine if there are medical factors, the most common being a side effect of medication, especially psychiatric medications.

The most typical cause is the man has developed an irrational fear of ejaculating within the vagina or in a woman's presence. The ejaculatory response has become self-conscious and inhibited. Men with ejaculatory inhibition believe there is something wrong, frightening, or immoral in letting go, feeling vulnerable, and abandoning themselves to sexual pleasure. Sex is a cooperative sharing between partners who are actively involved in giving and receiving pleasure. In ejaculatory inhibition, rather than orgasm being the natural culmination of an arousing experience, it becomes an anxiety-provoking goal he usually fails to achieve (and in some cases never achieves).

The most common technique problem is the man becomes quickly erect and didn't ask for additional stimulation. He reasons that since he's objectively aroused (has an erection), he feels silly delaying and engaging in erotic stimulation to enhance subjective arousal (feeling turned on). The problem is he maintains the same level—low to moderate arousal. The erotic flow toward higher levels of arousal and orgasm remains blocked.

A comfortable, involved, giving sexual partner is crucial in overcoming ejaculatory inhibition. A particular trap is the belief that a "real man" does not need the woman's cooperation and stimulation to heighten arousal and reach orgasm. The man mistakenly assumes he *should* be able to do it himself without making requests of his partner. He believes the myth that only "wimps" discuss sexual feelings or need erotic stimulation. As a man begins the aging process (in his thirties and continuing throughout his sexual life), he benefits from an intimate, interactive sexual relationship.

Other factors which cause ejaculatory inhibition include fear of being discovered while having sex, fear or misunderstanding of the vagina, a strict religious (and antisexual) upbringing, anxiety about ejaculation, aversion to one's semen, guilt over sexual pleasure, a traumatic sexual incident, fear of intimacy, or fear of pregnancy.

In middle-aged men, intermittent ejaculatory inhibition is associated with viewing marital sex as routine and unexciting. If a man expects not to reach a high degree of arousal with his wife, it becomes a self-fulfilling prophecy. The likelihood of this happening is especially great if he has not learned to make requests for the type of erotic stimulation which is most arousing. The man is used to automatic functioning and not needing stimulation. His lack of involvement makes it difficult to reach orgasm and is a sexual turnoff for the spouse. Sex becomes mechanical and mediocre. They are out of the rhythm of giving and receiving pleasure-oriented and erotic touching. It is not unusual for a man with intermittent ejaculatory inhibition to develop secondary erectile dysfunction and/or begin avoiding sexual encounters, which reinforces inhibited sexual desire.

Rather than ejaculatory inhibition being rare and difficult to treat, it is prevalent, has several variations, and is complex but understandable. Most important, it is changeable. The therapeutic strategy is to identify inhibitions and fears and develop sexual scenarios and techniques to overcome them. Some can be mastered, others modified so they don't interfere with the erotic flow, and others need to be accepted and worked around. The prime change strategies are to increase erotic stimulation and identify and use orgasm triggers. The couple works as an intimate team to increase comfort, eroticism, expressiveness, and to gain confidence that arousal will naturally culminate in orgasm.

Verbal and physical intimacy breaks down the walls of inhibition and sexual isolation. Involvement in the give-and-take of pleasuring and eroticism is key. Treatment strategies involve a one-two-three combination: being an intimate sexual team, comfort with pleasuring, and increased erotic stimulation. Even more important than sexual technique are changes in attitude (especially freedom to make sexual requests) and free emotional expression (letting go and experiencing high subjective arousal).

Jack

Men suffering from ejaculatory inhibition are an excellent example that to have a satisfying sexual relationship a person must learn to please himself as well as his partner. Jack, a client of Barry's, was a thirty-eight-year-old technical writer whose three children from two previous marriages lived with him. Jack functioned well psychologically, led an active life, enjoyed being a single father, and reported good relationships with women. He always experienced orgasm during masturbation, but ejaculated less than 10 percent of the time during partner sex. He consoled himself with the "blessing in disguise" theory that even though he was nonorgasmic, he was a good lover, and gave his partners orgasms. Jack felt it was unmanly to request stimulation. Instead, he focused on making sure he performed well, so she would have no cause to complain. As a result, he never got very sexually excited. As soon as he had an erection he initiated intercourse. Erection signifies a physiological readiness for intercourse, but Jack's subjective arousal (feeling turned on) was low. Jack felt "selfish" and "immature" requesting additional penile stimulation. He didn't allow himself to become an involved participant or feel highly aroused. Jack had made himself a "sexual servant" who was not entitled to enjoy sex for himself. Jack settled for orgasms during masturbation. He saw partner sex as for the woman, not him.

In therapy, Jack learned to request specific kinds of stimulation from his partner. He found oral stimulation particularly arousing when he was moving rather than being passive. Jack did not initiate intercourse until he was highly aroused, both subjectively and objectively. It was especially stimulating when his partner moved her pelvis in a circular manner during intercourse while simultaneously stroking and fondling his testicles. As he became confident making specific requests and gave himself permission to enjoy eroticism and let go, Jack experienced orgasm 75 percent of the time. Jack learned orgasm was the natural culmination of high levels of arousal and letting go.

STRATEGIES IN OVERCOMING EJACULATORY INHIBITION

The major strategy in treating a man with ejaculatory inhibition is to give him support and permission to enjoy pleasure and view ejaculation as a natural culmination of arousal. Like other sexual problems, the ideal is for the couple to see it as "their" problem rather than "his" problem and work together. They learn to be freer and more comfortable with sexual pleasure, being supportive, making sexual requests, and increasing eroticism. Even more important than sexual technique are changes in attitude, emotional expression, freedom to engage in give-and-take eroticism, and letting go emotionally and sexually. Treating ejaculatory inhibition is a gradual process of encouraging the man to be direct in requesting stimulation and experiencing and savoring erotic feelings. As he gains confidence and allows himself to be "selfish," high arousal will culminate in orgasm.

The two key techniques are requesting erotic (multiple) stimulation and being aware of orgasm triggers. Examples of multiple stimulation include using fantasy during partner sex, testicle stimulation during intercourse, stimulating your partner's breasts or anal area while she's stimulating you or kissing and stroking during intercourse. Her arousal increases your arousal. Orgasm triggers are very individualistic. Orgasm triggers can be identified during masturbation, where the man has more control. Examples of orgasm triggers include tensing leg and buttock muscles, increasing rhythm of thrusting, focusing on highly arousing fantasies, verbalizing you're "going to come."

Being comfortable ejaculating intravaginally is the goal, which needs to be approached in a stepwise manner. An important first step is to be comfortable ejaculating with the partner present. Lowering inhibitions and letting go by allowing yourself to ejaculate in front of your partner in response to her manual or oral stimulation is a positive step. If you are unable to do this, stimulate yourself to orgasm with your partner present, holding or caressing you. Enjoy eroticism, arousal and letting go. Subsequent steps include a pleasuring exercise where the man lies on his back, perhaps with a pillow under his head, with the woman sitting facing him with his legs over hers. She has easy contact with his body, especially genitals. He can stroke her thighs,

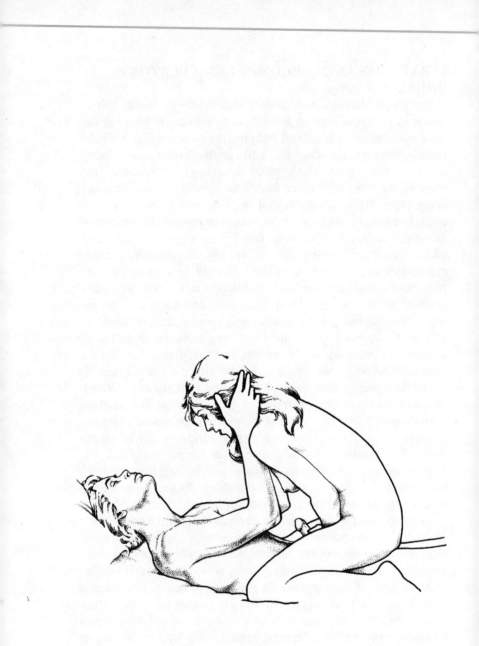

By utilizing multiple stimulation and fantasy, the man can overcome ejaculatory inhibition.

breasts, and vulva. She can experiment with mixing manual, oral, and rubbing stimulation to build a flow of pleasure, eroticism, and arousal. He can experiment with keeping his eyes open or closed, being passive or stroking her as she touches him, using erotic fantasy, being still or thrusting his pelvis, being silent or talking. Does sharing sexual feelings or fantasies increase or inhibit arousal? Awareness of what he needs to feel emotionally and sexually involved increases. He can be orgasmic with self-stimulation, rubbing his penis against her body or breasts, her manual stimulation, or fellatio.

In subsequent exercises, the emphasis is on the man making specific sexual requests, especially for multiple stimulation. The focus is on freer expression of sexual feelings. Examples include him kneeling over her so she can stroke him while he stimulates her and rubs his penis against her breasts. Or they stand in front of a mirror where visual stimulation adds an erotic dimension as he engages in oral breast stimulation and manual clitoral stimulation while she strokes his hair, penis, and testicles. Men find the woman's arousal heightens their arousal, facilitating erotic flow. He makes at least two erotic requests to enhance arousal. The requests can be verbal or conveyed by guiding—putting your hand over hers, moving your body toward her, or moving her body, hand, or mouth. You have a perfect right to make sexual requests. You might request stimulating her because as her arousal grows it increases your arousal. Make requests for multiple stimulation which can include asking her to tell you how turned on she feels as you lick her breasts or vulva, rub your penis between her legs or breasts while she's giving you anal stimulation, using sexual fantasies while touching and being touched, utilizing the range of sensory modalities—movement, sight, smell, touch, and sound.

A third set of exercises focus on orgasm triggers. Most men with ejaculatory inhibition are easily orgasmic during masturbation. That's because he is confident he'll be aroused and orgasmic. Being orgasmic is predictable, he has a sense of control and readiness to let go. He knows his "orgasm triggers" and is not self-conscious utilizing them. The man can become aware of his masturbatory orgasm triggers and transfer them to partner sex. Orgasm triggers are idiosyncratic. When approaching orgasm, some men stretch their legs or curl their toes; others make sounds or breath loudly and rapidly as they let go; some increase pelvic thrusting; others say "I'm coming now"; some imagine the culmination of their sexual fantasy and orgasm in reality as they fantasize orgasm. Be aware of your orgasm triggers. Some men find verbalizing triggers orgasm during partner sex. Some find it easier to be orgasmic with manual, oral, or rubbing stimulation, but most find intercourse their preferred mode to share orgasm. Men prefer man on top or rear entry, although woman on top and side by side have gained popularity because they facilitate multiple stimulation. Men who enjoy multiple (erotic) stimulation during nonintercourse sex find multiple stimulation during intercourse heightens eroticism and arousal.

Men with ejaculatory inhibition typically begin intercourse as soon as they get an erection. Don't initiate intercourse until you're highly aroused. Continue multiple stimulation during intercourse. The man is aware of and requests the type of intercourse stimulation that is most arousing. For example, the woman's slow and extended coital thrusting might be arousing for one man, while another might prefer she be passive while he moves in short, rapid strokes. There is a cultural myth that a man should only need intercourse stimulation. Perhaps that's true of twenty-year-old men, but it's not true for fifty-year-old men. Men in their thirties and forties would find intercourse more arousing if they engaged in multiple stimulation. As men age they want and need additional erotic stimulation. The most common form of multiple stimulation is fantasy—75 percent of males fantasize during intercourse. Fantasies are a bridge to heighten arousal. The man can enjoy and attend to all his feelings and sensations during intercourse.

Use the intercourse position which allows you the most stimulation and expressiveness. He controls coital thrusting and utilizes the type of intercourse movement (in-out, up-down, circular) and rhythm (long and slow, short and rapid) he finds most arousing. Many males enjoy testicle stimulation during intercourse, others prefer kissing and stroking the partner, others receiving anal stimulation.

No matter what intercourse position you use, be active and involved in giving and receiving pleasure. Be aware of what stimulation, in what sequence, and with what timing is most arousing. As arousal builds focus on feelings and sensations, request erotic stimulation, be aware of orgasm triggers, let go and allow arousal to flow to orgasm. The couple works together to reduce anxiety and inhibitions so he feels comfortable with intravaginal ejaculation. Remember, this is a joint effort. The couple develops a mutually satisfying sexual style in which arousal naturally culminates in orgasm.

Rather than trying to follow this program on their own, couples consult a sex therapist to help them learn or relearn freer, uninhibited attitudes, feelings, and behaviors. If the man does not have a regular sex partner, he might be particularly interested in consulting a therapist. Therapy not only helps him understand ejaculatory inhibition, but enables him to develop an individual program that will aid in reducing sexual anxiety and allow him to be freer emotionally and sexually.

HEALTHY ATTITUDES

As is true with other sexual problems, the man suffering from ejaculatory inhibition needs to take responsibility for his sexual behavior, accept the problem without feeling less masculine, and with the help and cooperation of his partner and/or a professional therapist work toward increased comfort, pleasure, and eroticism. It is important to note that, just as with erectile difficulty or early ejaculation, a man might experience ejaculatory inhibition as an occasional occurrence without it being a sign of sexual dysfunction. Any situation or feeling that interferes with free-flowing sexuality can block ejaculation. For instance, if he is tired, drank too much, is depressed, is angry with his partner, or if sex is interrupted by a phone call or children's demands, his urge to ejaculate is inhibited.

The problem of ejaculatory inhibition should not be confused with the normally occurring decrease of ejaculatory frequency in older men. As a man reaches sixty and beyond, he continues to enjoy intercourse, but feels less need to carry each encounter through to ejaculation. For instance, an older man who has intercourse five times a month may feel the need to ejaculate on only three or four of those occasions. Many older men (as well as women) do not understand this is a normal part of aging. They feel they're "over the hill" or have a sexual dysfunction. With aging, the importance of an intimate, interactive sexual relationship emphasizing pleasuring, variability, flexibility, and eroticism becomes more important. Being aware of and practicing this in your 40s and 50s is the best way to prevent ejaculatory inhibition.

Ejaculatory inhibition is neither a catastrophe nor something to be disregarded. It is a sexual dysfunction that, like other dysfunctions, is worth taking the time and effort to change. The challenge for the man is to break silence and isolation and ask his partner for increased intimacy, sharing, and eroticism. Ejaculatory inhibition responds to treatment. You owe it to yourself and your sexual relationship to reestablish comfort and confidence with pleasuring, eroticism, arousal and orgasm.

17

A COST-BENEFIT APPROACH TO EXTRAMARITAL SEX

Compared with the sexual vistas a single man is free to explore, marriage is a limited world. The ideal in marriage is sexual fidelity. For many men, raised on the belief sexual conquest is the means by which a man proves his masculinity, ignites desire, and provides excitement, being constrained to one woman for the rest of his life seems unacceptable. Even when he has no intention of engaging in extramarital sex, he finds himself toying with thoughts of a forbidden affair. An affair is a way to demonstrate he's a "real man," not a wimp constrained by marital bonds. Sooner or later, the chance to engage in extramarital sex will arise since such opportunities are readily available, especially in our urban, anonymous culture. Since a "real man" never turns down a sexual opportunity, an extramarital affair appears predestined, regardless of whether he actively pursues it or tries to avoid it.

MAKING CHOICES ABOUT EXTRAMARITAL SEX

Such a fatalistic attitude deprives you of the power to make choices and take responsibility for your behavior. In the case of extramarital sex, these choices can have far-reaching consequences. Thinking about your values and feelings regarding marital sexuality and extramarital affairs, and making decisions that are in your best interest is extremely important. It is worthwhile to consider extramarital sex in a thoughtful manner, distinguish among the different levels of extramarital involvement, and

231

weigh the advantages and disadvantages for you as a person and for your marriage.

Don't be controlled by ready-made opinions and cultural stereotypes, whether radical or traditional in origin. Each exerts its own tyranny over our thinking. The traditional attitude is an extramarital affair, if discovered, is sufficient cause for ending the marriage. The offended spouse leaves or forces the other to leave and all communication between them ceases, except that carried out through lawyers. There is a different commonly accepted traditional idea: the husband is expected to have brief clandestine affairs, but the wife will remain strictly faithful and prefers not to "really know" about his affairs. The premarital double standard transferred to extramarital sexuality.

Radical couples propose an entirely different framework. An idea which gained currency some years ago was it is not extramarital sex but sexual exclusivity that is the enemy of marriage. Monogamy restricts the individual's ability to express himself and relate freely. The ideal marriage is one in which neither partner questions how the other spends his time or with whom. According to this view, people are naturally polygamous. So "co-marital affairs," threesomes, mate swapping, group sex—including bisexuality—can be comfortably incorporated within the marital context, provided both partners give up "selfish, old-fashioned feelings of jealousy and possessiveness." Extramarital sex is not a threat but an opportunity to liberate both people and achieve freedom and openness.

If we look carefully at traditional and radical attitudes, it becomes clear they are equally doctrinaire, equally unsuitable as guides for real-life behavior. To see how emotional and value laden they are, we have only to look at the contrasting terminology. Those who are opposed to affairs use terms such as *adultery, cheating on your wife, being unfaithful.* Those who favor extramarital sex, prefer terms such as *personal and sexual sharing, not being hung-up by jealousy,* and *open marriage.* To the extent possible, we will attempt to avoid value-laden terms and doctrinaire attitudes. We try to take an objective and constructive approach to the issue of extramarital sex. There is no blanket judgment—good or bad—that can apply to all people and all extramarital affairs. Rather, each affair must be considered in the context of its meaning for the individual and his marriage. The individual's and the couple's religious and personal values must be carefully considered.

TYPES OF AFFAIRS

For the purpose of analysis, it is helpful to separate extramarital affairs into three categories: (1) the high opportunity-low involvement affair, (2) the ongoing affair, and (3) the comparison affair. The high opportunity-low involvement encounter is the most common type for men. It may occur during an out of town business trip or as a pickup at a bar or party. Although the desire for an exciting, illicit experience or for sexual variety plays a part, the main reason casual encounters happen is that it is possible for them to happen. The opportunity presents itself and there seem to be few liabilities in accepting it. Often, these are paid experiences with prostitutes or at massage parlors. The man wants a sexual activity his wife is unwilling to engage in or, just as likely, he's uncomfortable asking her for. Most commonly, this is fellatio. It is common for the married clients of prostitutes to request oral sex rather than intercourse.

There are advantages as well as disadvantages to the high opportunity-low involvement encounter. One advantage is since there is little or no emotional attachment, it is the least disruptive to the marriage. A man may feel guilt as a result of anonymous sex, but, for most men, it's not likely to compete on an emotional level with his marital relationship. If his wife discovers the affair, she may feel less threatened than she would by a serious involvement. It is possible for the sexual encounter to enhance his sexual repertoire. He learns new techniques or acquires an enthusiasm for sex that can transfer into the marriage. It provides sexual pleasure if he receives little satisfaction from marital sex, as well as adds an element of excitement and adventure to his life.

The disadvantages of the casual encounter include those that exist for unmarried men as well—the danger of sexually transmitted diseases and/or pregnancy. The new danger, especially with prostitutes, is transmission of HIV/AIDS. Although HIV is considerably more difficult to transmit female to male, it is possible. So safer sex, specifically, use of the condom, is strongly recommended at *each* sexual encounter.

People who meet casually for sex seldom bother discussing health issues or contraceptive methods. The man assumes she is on the pill or he doesn't care, the result can be an unwanted pregnancy. There is the possibility the woman has an STD, and if the encounter is truly anonymous she may not be concerned about infecting him. The rate of STDs is highest in casual affairs and among prostitutes. If the man does contract an STD, he is likely to give it to his wife. He then faces the extremely embarrassing task of having to reveal the affair so he can alert her to the need for medical treatment. Another disadvantage is the man becomes involved in the drinking and drug culture that revolves around bars and prostitution.

A further disadvantage is while providing sexual novelty, it detracts from the marital relationship. The casual encounter reinforces the double standard approach to sex. A man who finds his sexual excitement and variety outside the marriage has diminished motivation to improve marital sex. There is the danger that casual encounters or visits to massage parlors will become a habit, reinforcing the dichotomy of marital sex as routine and extramarital sex as charged and adventurous. This not only sells short the potential for pleasure in marriage, but contributes to its deterioration.

THE ONGOING AFFAIR

The ongoing affair is the second most common form of extramarital sex for men. These affairs are based on an understanding that the man and woman will meet periodically for sex, conversation, drinks or dinner, but little else. There is no expectation the relationship will develop, grow more serious or intimate. Possessiveness is discouraged by one or both partners. Examples are the salesman who spends an evening with a particular woman each time business brings him to her area of the country, the man who visits a divorced woman once a week for a sexual liaison, the executive who is having an affair with his secretary. These affairs are usually of short duration, but if they satisfy the needs of both parties and if carried on without fear of detection, may continue for years.

The ongoing affair has definite advantages. It allows for continuity and human contact and provides a supplemental sexual outlet. At the same time, it does not require a major emotional commitment or the expenditure of time or energy. It allows the man to talk about ideas, frustrations, and emotions he does not share with his wife. The affair furnishes not only a sexual release but a psychological one as well. If the man's marriage is irredeemable, yet he does not wish to divorce, this type of affair helps him maintain appearances. The ongoing affair assuages loneliness as well as meets sexual needs. This relationship, though it might settle into a familiar routine, can, at the same time, create a sense of adventure. The experience of arranging a secret rendezvous, of leading a clandestine and illicit "double life," provides a certain charm and excitement.

The ongoing affair has the same disadvantages as the casual encounter—the possibilities of detection, pregnancy and STDs/HIV—as well as some of its own. The greatest danger is it may lead to a deeper, more personal involvement than expected. Emotions are unpredictable, there is no guarantee they will remain at the level intended for them. Such unexpected emotional involvement may be mutual or one-sided. In either case, it leads to unanticipated complications.

People's lives are not geared to handling sudden emotional overloads. The consequences of being caught between a demanding, jealous mistress and an increasingly suspicious wife may be disastrous. This type of affair consumes more time and psychological energy than anticipated, detracting from other areas of a man's life. One of the first effects is on the relationship with his children; he simply does not have the time to devote to being a parent. He has less time for business, hobbies, and friends. Ironically, what was originally undertaken for pleasure and recreation ends up increasing the demands and restrictions on his time and energy. Unless the man manages to break off the affair (usually an immensely harder and more complex task than starting it), the situation may get out of control and end in catastrophe.

Another disadvantage is the loss of intimacy with his wife. Not only does the affair have a negative effect on marital sex, it is likely to affect emotional intimacy as well. The man puts less energy into his marriage and shares his thoughts and feelings less. Because of guilt and/or fear of discovery, he is guarded or uncommunicative. His wife may become suspicious or feel he no longer cares about her. She withdraws intimacy and affection, causing him to turn more and more to the affair. He feels lonely and emotionally needy, dissatisfied and vulnerable.

Brian and Ellen

Brian and Ellen provide a good example of the toll a husband's extramarital affairs can take in terms of the time and energy they consume. It was Ellen who sought individual therapy. She was unhappy, dispirited, complaining the responsibilities of caring for a home and two children left her feeling inadequate. She felt a need to change her life and was considering returning to school. It soon became clear one of her main problems was marital, Brian was too distracted to provide practical help or emotional support. At the therapist's suggestion, Ellen requested Brian participate in the therapy sessions. After talking to them together and Brian alone, the story behind their present troubles emerged.

Brian was a leasing agent with flexible hours and contact with a wide variety of people. During the first two years of marriage their sex life had been good, but after Ellen became pregnant sexual relations stopped almost completely. Brian engaged in three casual affairs. The most common time for a man to begin an extramarital affair is during his wife's first pregnancy. He found extramarital sex more exciting than ''settled-down'' marital sex. Brian felt he'd recaptured the feelings and challenge he experienced before marriage. He enjoyed getting away with something by keeping the affairs secret. Brian continued this pattern until, after the birth of their second child five years later, things became too much. Between his job, wife, children, and the intricate circle of extramarital connections, he was living life too fast with too little time. Brian's life was chaotic, and Ellen was suffering as much as he. As these problems were explored during therapy, they realized their marital bond was broken. The best way of dealing with the stress was to dissolve the marriage. There was simply too much anger, disappointment, and alienation on both sides to devote the necessary energy to rebuild the marriage.

COMPARISON AFFAIRS

The third category of affairs is the most complex as well as the most threatening to the status quo: the sexually intimate, emotionally involving comparison affair. More of the man's emotional and sexual needs are met by the affair than his marriage. There are definite advantages as well as disadvantages in the comparison affair.

An intimate affair can be a powerful ego boost, particularly for someone who is feeling down about a job, family problems, or middle-age blues. Love, excitement, and passion had been missing from his life, and it is exhilarating to feel them again. Finding he is capable of loving and being loved gives him a new lease on life. It has been said that love is the best tonic, and this can be true of an extramarital relationship. A comparison affair can have a profound regenerative effect. It may galvanize the man into confronting issues he felt little motivation to address. For example, if a man's marriage has deteriorated beyond repair and he has been too apathetic to do anything about it, a comparison affair shows him what he's missing and spurs him to get a divorce. In fact, the single most frequent cause of a man leaving his marriage is a comparison affair.

The potential disadvantages of a comparison affair, however, are also great. The dangers and problems associated with the other two types of affairs result from this type as well. In addition, the comparison affair has the most potential for ending disastrously. It places the greatest psychological stress on the man, since in effect he is leading two lives. One of the two women will end up feeling hurt and rejected, and there is the possibility he'll lose both relationships. The emotional conflict can become intense, and have a wrenching effect on family, job, and sense of well-being. Most men are incapable of sustaining a double life, no matter what one reads in the spate of books and articles advising people how to deal with multiple love relationships. Men who become involved in a comparison affair eventually have to choose between the affair and the marriage. This choice is accompanied by considerable turmoil and psychological pain. The joke in mental health circles is if people stopped having affairs it would cut business by one-third. Comparison affairs throw marriages into crisis when discovered, and even if not discovered cause emotional turmoil.

A subcategory of the comparison affair is the highly romantic, emotionally intense relationship that has not been sexually consummated. The sense of the forbidden and the tantalizing fantasy of being sexual controls the man's thoughts. Discussions about how they are just best friends and shouldn't get involved sexually serves to build sexual tension. In this atmosphere, a kiss or touch ignites powerful feelings and desires. Unconsummated affairs are as powerful a threat to a marriage as a consummated affair.

TAKING RESPONSIBILITY FOR DECISIONS

There is a good deal of simplification in this discussion. In real life an extramarital encounter is unique and does not fit neatly into any category. No matter how carefully we enumerate the pros and cons of an action, we can never balance one side against the other in a truly objective way. We choose intuitively and on the spur of the moment, often regretting this. That is all the more reason for taking stock of our situation, feelings, and values so we have a basis for future decisions. Ideally, a husband and wife, early in their marriage, would frankly discuss the issue of extramarital sex to share and clarify their thoughts and feelings. In reality, this is seldom, if ever, done. The husband usually has an implicit assumption that is different from the spouse's. The man assumes his wife won't have an affair and he might have a high opportunity encounter or an ongoing affair. Few people plan to have a comparison affair.

OUR PERSONAL EXPERIENCE

When Emily and Barry married, part of the traditional, male chauvinist baggage Barry brought into the relationship was the assumption he could have high opportunity affairs. He hadn't thought about Emily's expectations, but assumed she would not have an affair. After a few months of marriage the subject came up, and Emily told Barry she would not accept a double standard approach to extramarital sex. One of the goals in our relationship was to develop and maintain a sense of equity. Barry assured Emily the only affair he would consider would be high opportunity-low involvement; an affair would be nonemotional and kept totally apart from the marriage. She said if he could have affairs she would reserve the right to have an affair. Emily expressed her distaste for casual affairs, if she had an affair it would be emotionally involving. We discussed whether we were comfortable with this, and Barry admitted he wasn't. We confronted the issue of whether we could tolerate a sexual double standard in our marriage. It seemed clear that, in our case at least, a single standard would be healthier. A commitment to not have affairs was a better choice for us.

We made our feelings and expectations explicit. The advantage is our agreement allows us freedom to travel and interact with opposite sex friends without worrying about the spouse's commitment. It also makes us more vulnerable to hurt if either breaks the agreement and has an affair. If this did occur, it would cause disappointment and anger and would require a good deal of talking and confrontation, but because of our strong commitment, would not devastate our marriage. This agreement has met our needs, but this does not mean it would be good for you or your marriage. Be aware of your values, feelings, experiences, and life situation.

GUIDELINES ABOUT AFFAIRS

The first guideline is the better the marriage, the less there is to be gained from an affair. If a basically good relationship is beset with sexual or emotional problems, it makes more sense to work on the problems together rather than form a new attachment and, in effect, resolve them unilaterally. If the problems seem overwhelming, then a marital or sex therapist can be consulted. Many people reject the idea of seeking professional help because they see it as a sign of weakness, an acknowledgment that things have gotten beyond their capacity to deal with. But, if anything, the decision to consult a professional is an indication of a couple's commitment, a sign of the value they place on their marriage. A therapist with training and experience in dealing with marital and sexual problems can provide the objective viewpoint and knowledge needed to understand and resolve conflicts.

Beware of self-deception in extramarital affairs. It is easy to convince yourself that what you are doing is motivated by the best intentions when it is not. For example, where extramarital sex is concerned, honesty is not necessarily the best policy. Confessing an affair may appear to be a virtuous act. You claim to be promoting an honest, open marital relationship, but what you may actually be doing is expressing hostility and/or trying to alleviate your guilt. Living with the discomfort caused by keeping a part of your life secret may be the price you pay for an affair. It is unfair to expect a spouse to accept the affair and go on with the marriage as if nothing happened. Having an affair and enjoying a state of innocence is too much to expect. One strategy, persuading your wife to have an affair to "even things up"—is a form of coercion that reflects the husband's need to assuage his guilt more than concern for his wife. An affair might be a diversionary and dishonest way of expressing a desire to split up the marriage.

Some patterns indicate the motivation behind the affair is destructive. For example, the man who has a series of affairs, usually with younger women, in an attempt to prove his attractiveness and sexual prowess. He may tell himself his wife no longer turns him on, forcing him to seek sexual gratification elsewhere, but there is a basic problem he refuses to face.

Sexual dysfunction is a poor reason to seek extramarital sex. Men (and women) with a sexual dysfunction have an affair to see if they are functional (that is, does he have ejaculatory control, a strong erection, greater desire, or absence of ejaculatory inhibition?). But, once you have that information the issue still is how to deal with marital sex. A more honest and productive approach would be to address the problem by seeking sex therapy.

Another example of a destructive pattern is the man who seeks extramarital encounters with married neighbors, his wife's friends, coworkers, and others whose identity would make detection both extremely likely and extremely painful. He's using extramarital sex as a means of inflicting punishment on either himself or his wife—and possibly on both.

Extramarital sex can serve a positive role in the man's life. Like a premarital affair, an extramarital affair can be a learning experience; it shows a man what is possible in a relationship, sexually, emotionally or both. Whether the knowledge gained in extramarital sex is used to enrich the marriage or hasten its dissolution is a matter the individual must choose for himself.

Jack

Jack, an older student in Barry's human sexual behavior course, wrote a personal sex history as part of a class assignment. His story illustrates the positive effects of extramarital sex. Jack was a twenty-nine-year-old accountant who had grown up in a religious fundamentalist home. He married at twenty-one, and had not had sex with anyone besides his wife. Jack was happy with his job, house, and particularly his four-year-old son, but he felt his life lacked excitement. Marital sex was functional, but routine. Although it took two years to admit it, he wanted an affair. It took another six months before the opportunity arose at an out of town business meeting.

Although sex that first night was not great, Jack felt tremendously free and liberated. During the next year, he sought opportunities to travel and have sexual liaisons. One woman introduced him to oral sex. Jack initiated his wife into experimenting with oral-genital sex. After a year, Jack encouraged his wife to have an affair to "free her up sexually." They made an agreement not to talk about the details of their affairs, but to share sexual scenarios and techniques. This pattern continued for two years, and their sex life prospered.

At present Jack has no affairs since marital sex has improved and there had been emotionally draining discussions and arguments, especially regarding Jack's reactions to his wife's two affairs. However, if a really tempting sexual opportunity presents itself when he's out of town, he would find it difficult to turn down. Their marital relationship has matured, due to talking about their emotional and sexual feelings. Efforts to incorporate techniques learned in extramarital relationships brought them closer and helped reduce the doubts and fears that accompany affairs.

SWINGING AND OPEN MARRIAGE

People claim "swinging," the mutual exchange of sex partners, is one way to have extramarital sex without endangering the marital relationship. One to three percent of married couples have experimented with swinging. The assertion is that by having extramarital affairs under controlled conditions, you inject variety and excitement into the marriage while maintaining trust. There is nothing inherently destructive or deviant about swinging—it depends on the couple, their goals, values, and the nature of the relationship. It is worth noting, however, that few couples swing for more than six months. It is usually the husband who is responsible for making the decision to swing and for calling it off.

"Open marriage," an arrangement in which each partner is free to have extramarital relationships without hiding these activities, has been advocated in bestselling books. However, research on open marriage strongly indicates it is not a viable model for most couples. It's an example of something that sounds good as cocktail party chatter, but has negative effects on people's lives and relationships. There is a great potential for coercion and self-deception. The assumption is a mature and liberated person would not feel anger nor jealousy about his spouse being sexual with another man. Since all of us want to believe we are mature and liberated, we deny negative reactions toward our partner's extramarital relationships when, in fact, we feel them. The danger comes when these suppressed feelings burst forth, capsizing the marriage in a storm of resentment and violent emotion.

REACTIONS TO YOUR WIFE'S EXTRAMARITAL AFFAIR

Statistically, a man is more likely to engage in extramarital sex than a woman. The estimate is 30 percent of married men have at least one extramarital encounter. Between 15 and 20 percent of wives have extramarital sex.[14] A prime factor is men have more opportunities for sex outside of marriage. Freedom to have affairs is part of the male role. In addition, males are more likely to engage in paid sex, which is very unusual for women. Another factor is men are less experienced than women at turning down sex. A man should learn to apply logic and understanding not only to his real or potential involvements, but to those of his wife.

Men react more strongly to their wives' extramarital affairs than women do to their husbands'. This is due, in part, to the double standard. It is considered more acceptable for a man to have extramarital sex, but a woman who has an affair is regarded as unfaithful and dishonest. This reaction reflects the kind of affairs women have—the most typical female affair is a comparison affair. The casual encounter (high opportunity-low involvement) is rarer among women. This reflects the profound and complex differences in cultural conditioning affecting male-female sexual attitudes and behavior. There is support, if not outright peer pressure, for men to engage in casual affairs, which is not true of female peer groups. Typically, the woman has an affair to fulfill emotional and/or sexual needs unsatisfied in the marriage. The wife's affair is significant in terms of its implications for marital intimacy and stability. This is another reason men find their wives' affair threatening.

There is no pat strategy for dealing with the discovery of a wife's extramarital affair. However, here are practical guidelines that might be of value. The traditional masculine role when a man discovers his wife is having an affair is to respond with vindictive rage and possibly violence. This is destructive and to be avoided. The mistaken belief is to react in any other way compromises his honor and masculinity. The fact your wife is having an affair need not be interpreted as an insult to your masculinity. Nor is it a sign the marriage is destined to end in divorce. However, it does mean the marriage is in major trouble. It probably means important personal and/or sexual needs are not being met by the marriage.

The best way to understand your wife's affair is to assess its significance in the context of the marital relationship. The affair may be, at least partially, a message drawing attention to marital deficits. Her decision to have an affair may reflect boredom and dissatisfaction with her roles as wife, mother, worker, and social organizer. It may be an expression of frustration that you do not devote enough time and attention, she feels neglected and unappreciated. It may reflect anger that you do not treat her as an equitable partner. Two common reasons for female affairs are greater opportunity and the affair as a statement of personal independence.

Men are threatened by the idea their wife has greater sexual satisfaction with another man. This fear is heightened if there is a sexual problem in the marriage. In the majority of cases, however, it is the need for emotional and psychological satisfaction that motivates women to have affairs, not the desire for better sex. The question the man needs to ask is not "How have I failed as a sex partner?" but rather "What emotional and sexual needs have I not satisfied as a husband and lover?"

On the other hand, don't make the mistake of interpreting your wife's affair egocentrically, as though whatever she did could only have significance in terms of yourself. Sometimes an affair has to do with opportunity. Sometimes it is the woman's way of dealing with depression or boredom, or to prove she is attractive and desirable. Sometimes relationships deteriorate to the level they cannot be repaired. The message conveyed by the wife's affair may not be that she wants more love and attention from you, but she has decided to leave the marriage and the affair is a transition step. Then, of course, there is the possibility she has fallen in love with another man—not a pleasant turn of events, but one that must be faced and dealt with. A marriage ended by an affair is particularly hard on a male, but he can be a survivor and rebuild his personal and sexual self-esteem.

CLOSING THOUGHTS

If we view marriage as an important relationship that can provide great rewards for the couple willing to work at enhancing the quality of their marital bond, then we regard extramarital sex with wariness. In most cases, the effect of an extramarital affair on a marriage is negative. For the man or woman who is dissatisfied with marriage, either sexually, emotionally or both, it is more profitable to work at solving these problems than to seek escape in a second relationship and leave the marriage hanging. In and of themselves, extramarital affairs cannot be categorically judged as either bad or good, but must be understood according to how they affect each individual and the marriage. In certain cases, extramarital affairs may have a positive influence on a marriage, and in other cases may serve a useful purpose in a flawed marital relationship. A man thinking about engaging in extramarital sex should keep in mind there is always an element of risk, personally and maritally.

18
SINGLE AGAIN: DIVORCE AND WIDOWERS

Some radical theorists have suggested the laws governing marriage should be changed to conform to those that apply in business dealings. Instead of marriage being a permanent commitment and putting all your security, finances, and sexuality into the marriage, you would sign a contract that specified limits, especially financial, and what would happen if the marriage failed. There would be a time limit—say, five years—after which the marriage contract could be renewed, modified, or terminated.

Such arrangements may indeed become popular with divorced people. However, most men marry with the expectation, or at least the hope, that this relationship will be a source of intimacy and security for a lifetime. How many of us achieve this goal, however, is another matter.

A substantial proportion of today's marriages fail to live up to "happily ever after." Out of every ten couples choosing wedlock, approximately half will end in divorce.[15] Although divorce is very common in our culture (the U.S. has the highest divorce rate of any industrialized nation) and is less stigmatized than in the past, the transition to being single again is difficult. It takes energy and effort to adjust psychologically, socially, and sexually. Research studies indicate the psychological process of deciding to divorce, going through the divorce, and accepting the reality of divorce takes at least two years.

In the 1950s, unless there was a clear and overwhelming reason to divorce (spouse or child abuse, alcoholism, lack of financial support), couples stayed together. There was strong family, community, and religious support for marriage. Dysfunctional

245

and destructive marriages continued because it was the easy thing to do. In the 1990s, when one or both spouses feel the marital bond is unsatisfactory or broken, the marriage ends. Not only is there a high rate of divorce, but the number of women leaving their husbands has dramatically increased. Approximately 70 percent of divorces are initiated by women. Thus, the man has to deal with being the one who is left rather than the leaver.

The single again man must learn to accept the loss of an accustomed companion and sexual partner. No matter how poor the relationship, divorce leaves an emotional gap that is a source of pain and grief for months. He must consider the options available now that he is single again and think through alternatives.

A divorced man may experience considerable depression, based as much on a sense of failure as a feeling of loss. Divorced men believe they are failures in the eyes of family, friends, and society—they have not lived up to the husband/father roles. Rather than dwell on this sense of defeat, it is far more productive to view a divorce as an unfortunate but necessary step, one that can ultimately be a valuable learning experience. If it is not possible for partners to achieve satisfaction within the marriage, then divorce is a logical and psychologically healthy alternative. Men report feeling relieved to be free of an unsatisfying marriage. The lessons a man can learn from divorce, about himself and the nature of marriage, can be helpful in dealing with future relationships. The psychologically healthiest approach is to view the divorce as a learning experience and being single again as a challenge and new opportunity.

CHILD CUSTODY AND VISITATION

The man with children has to deal with his role as father, including child-support payments and visitation rights. This complex subject could be a book in itself, but we can offer basic guidelines. Children often blame themselves for the divorce—they mistakenly believe if they had behaved differently the marriage might have been saved. Make it clear the problem lay not with the children or your role as parent, but with the relationship between yourself and your ex-wife. Divorce is an adult decision and responsibility. It is important to stress the children need not take sides. Although the marriage has ended, you are still their father and care about them. You will remain integrally involved in their lives.

Maintaining financial responsibilities to your children, no matter what your feelings about your ex-wife, is important for their sense of trust and well-being. Unfortunately, mothers are given custody much more often than fathers. We are strong supporters of the concept of joint custody, when feasible. No matter what the custody arrangement, it is important to be consistent and caring during visitation with your children.

There is a good deal of anger and bitterness between ex-spouses, and often they use the children as the battleground. This is destructive not only for children but subverts your ability to develop a new life. Although you are likely to be angry, or at least highly ambivalent, toward the ex-spouse, for your sake and the children's sake everything would go better if each of you succeeded in establishing a new life. Seldom do ex-spouses remain friendly, that's an unrealistic expectation. Relate to each other in a respectful, cooperative manner and deal only with child-rearing issues. Keep emotional distance, especially regarding new relationships. You couldn't influence the ex-spouse when you were married, so why would you think you could influence her when divorced.

NEW RELATIONSHIPS

It can be both too easy and too difficult for a recently divorced man to establish a new relationship. Particularly when the divorce involved a great deal of emotional pain, he might be unwilling to become intimate with another woman and make himself vulnerable to further hurt. Still, most men find the dangers of investing in a relationship are outweighed by the joy and satisfaction a new relationship can bring. In fact, five out of six divorced men do remarry, typically within three years after the divorce. What happens all too frequently, however, is the man picks a new partner who is remarkably similar to the ex-wife and with whom the tensions and difficulties of the first marriage are repeated. Or, he goes to the other extreme and chooses someone totally different and discovers she lacks crucial traits he needs in a spouse.

The divorce rate for second marriages is higher than for first marriages. Instead of falling into this trap, make every effort to use the unsuccessful marriage as an opportunity to learn what elements must be present to make a viable, satisfying marriage. The man who wishes to remarry should take time to seek out a truly compatible partner rather than rush into marriage to escape loneliness or prove something to himself or the ex-spouse. When a man uses divorce as an opportunity for learning, his second marriage will be intimate and satisfying. Men in stable second marriages value their marriages more than men in first marriages.

Jim

Jim was a divorced man of thirty-two whose first marriage lasted three years. Although the divorce was bitter and drawn out, Jim continued to function well through the turmoil, completing a master's degree in business administration. During the waiting period, Jim had a series of affairs lasting a few weeks each. When the divorce became final, he decided he'd had enough of short sexually-oriented contacts and wanted a serious relationship, though not necessarily one that would evolve to marriage.

After two unsuccessful tries, he established a close relationship with a divorced woman with a young child. They lived together for two and a half years. When the time came to decide whether to marry, Jim decided this was a better living-together relationship than it would be a marriage. Jim wanted to marry only if it were an up-front commitment and he were sure this was a viable bond. That relationship would have been backing into a marginal marriage, and although it was hard, Jim left.

Jim met Judy at work and they began dating after three months. Judy was divorced and had two children. Although their relationship became intimate, Jim continued to live alone, having learned the dangers of establishing a living-together situation without first being clear about what was involved. Jim wanted to be sure he remained in the relationship for healthy reasons, not because he needed to escape the dating scene, avoid lonely nights, or have someone take care of him. Jim and Judy decided to live together after eight months. Six months later they married, but not before thoroughly discussing their expectations and commitment. They agreed Jim would adopt her two children and in a year would have a child of their own. They discussed sexual feelings, finances, career plans, child rearing and living arrangements, making sure in each case the problems which had occurred in their first marriages would not be repeated. This planning paid off. Their marriage is solid and satisfying.

SOCIAL FRIENDSHIPS

Before establishing a relationship, a divorced man must be able to meet appropriate women. Our society does not make this easy. Married people tend to have married friends, and a newly divorced man finds the social occasions open to him are reduced. Some married couples, unaware of his loneliness, feel awkward about including him in their activities. Rather than expecting others to read his mind, he should take responsibility for letting friends know his needs and feelings. They may be uncomfortable discussing social possibilities and women with him, or unsure whether or how to bring up his divorce. Some go to the other extreme and assume he is having a great sexual time as a bachelor and tell him how much they envy him. It is up to him to be honest and tell them how he is doing and what he needs or doesn't need. He must make clear whether he objects to being invited to gatherings where his ex-wife might be present, whether he appreciates his friends' efforts to "match him up," and whether he is comfortable being a single person at couple get-togethers.

SEXUAL FRIENDSHIPS AND DEGREES OF INTIMACY

One of the first questions to ask yourself is what level of intimacy are you interested in. Some men are principally interested in picking someone up at a bar or party and having a one-night stand. Often the motivation is to reassert one's sexuality. It's a way of saying you're an attractive male who can enjoy sex with a variety of women. This is a transitory phase that soon grows stale.

The concept of a sexual friendship is appealing for many men. This involves establishing a companionable relationship that allows for communication, emotional intimacy, and sexual sharing, but without the implicit promise this will be a permanent union. It has the advantages of friendship, without the promises of marriage, permanence, or deep levels of trust and intimacy. Some sexual friendships include an agreement about exclusive dating and/or sexual exclusivity, but many do not. A sexual friendship might last two months or two years. Many continue to be friends after stopping being a sexual couple. Men look back on a sexual friendship and feel good about the relationship, their time together, and themselves. Others find the end of the relationship leaves a bad taste; there are hurt feelings and a sense of being "ripped off" or "taken for a ride." This is most likely to happen when the man (or woman) has unrealistic expectations, makes promises he can't keep, or tries to make the relationship more than it can be. For example, couples who move in together—or even worse, buy a house together or switch jobs or cities for the sake of the relationship—feel cheated and bitter. A common trap is for the man to become overly involved with the woman's children or for her to become a "temporary stepmother" for his children. Enjoy the sexual friendship for what it is. Keep a realistic perspective on the degree of intimacy, trust, and permanence this relationship can offer. A marriage should never be more than one-third of self-esteem; a sexual friendship is an important but transitory part of your life and should never be more than 15 percent of self-esteem. One does not make major life changes for a sexual friendship.

What about the man who is looking for intimacy and security and wants to find a marriage partner? First, be sure you are doing this for positive reasons—you are aware how to make a healthy choice and are ready to make the emotional and sexual commitment necessary to sustain a successful marriage. It's not worth marrying unless this relationship adds significantly to your life. You can live a fulfilling and satisfying life as a single person. Marrying to alleviate loneliness, have a mother for your children, or someone to take care of you, is likely to backfire and cause more disruption than remaining single. The decision to share your life with a spouse is to enhance emotional and sexual intimacy and maintain a secure bond.

A crucial guideline is to clearly and realistically discuss issues with the woman, don't marry out of romantic love or desperation. Some men are so eager to marry they make all kinds of assumptions about their new partner. Rather than being swept away by romantic illusions or an unrealistic belief this relationship is perfect, ask yourself and your partner the hard and important questions about a second marriage. What is your life plan for the next five years? What are the special issues—sexuality, living arrangements, careers, finances, stepchildren, whether to have additional children, dealing with family and friends—that need to be discussed and agreements reached? Especially important is awareness of the issues that were problematic in the first marriage—whether sex, finances, arguing in destructive ways, spending time together, or extramarital affairs. View them as "traps" to monitor and avoid in this marriage. Rather than ignoring the sensitive areas and hoping they won't recur, disclose them to your partner. If they cause difficulties, attend to them immediately. As the folk saying goes, "An ounce of prevention is worth a pound of cure." If you value this marriage and want it to be emotionally and sexually successful, devote the time and psychological energy to attend to these issues and problem-solve in a respectful, cooperative manner.

BEING A WIDOWER

The death of a spouse is a severe trauma for the survivor. It is normal to experience strong emotions. In cases where the death was sudden, the husband's first—and natural—reaction is to reject the situation as unreal, to feel it can't be happening. Whether we realized it or not, a spouse fills a very large space in our lives. To have that presence removed without warning leaves a gulf we are incapable of comprehending at first. It can take months before the widower feels he is part of the world again. Especially for men under fifty, the idea of being a widower is foreign. There are many more women who become widows than men who are widowers. Yet, the reality is you're a widower. This needs to be accepted and dealt with, not denied.

The next reaction is one of grief and depression. As the widower begins to take in the dimensions of his loss, feelings of sadness seem overwhelming. At times he may find himself crying uncontrollably or experiencing a breakdown of self-control. Although this is contrary to the traditional male image, accept this as natural and important in the grieving process. Painful, often maudlin, feelings and regrets disturb him. He thinks about things he and his wife had planned to do and now will never have the chance. He may feel guilty for not being more attentive or generous, for not buying gifts or taking her places. He may even feel guilty because he is the survivor and can continue to enjoy life while she is dead. Anger is not an uncommon reaction. Many widowers feel furious at their wives for abandoning them, for leaving them alone—an irrational but natural feeling. Feeling angry with a dead spouse does not mean you hated her; it is a sign of how important she was and how hard it is to accept her loss. You're angry at the need to reestablish your life as a single man. Anger is part of the grieving process.

PRACTICAL ISSUES FACING THE WIDOWER

Marriage involves not only emotional ties but practical considerations as well. Much of the distress a widower experiences is connected with feeling overwhelmed with the responsibilities that are suddenly his alone. This is especially true when there are children to take care of. The widower feels it is unfair that he must do all the things he and his wife once shared, especially caring for the children's physical and emotional needs and running the household on a day-to-day basis. There is a temptation for the grief-stricken man to shut these responsibilities out by ignoring them or drinking heavily. It is important to step up to issues rather than deny them. Recognize the problems that exist and face them head-on rather than avoiding. He is entitled to his grief, but in the midst of grief he must deal with the present reality, which includes responsibilities to his children. He must begin to plan for the future and rebuild his life.

Men find it very difficult to take full responsibility for home and family. One alternative is to ask a female friend or relative with whom he feels comfortable to help him manage. Having someone who is familiar with the running of a household will make it easier for the widower to live on his own. He should not reject help when offered on the grounds that he must be self-sufficient. It is not a sign of weakness to accept help while adjusting to the loss of a spouse. You are not seeking to establish a dependency, but to use the person's support to help you act in a responsible way. It is a sign of your commitment to reorganizing your life and family.

It is very helpful if the widower has someone with whom he can share his complex feelings of guilt, sadness, anger, and worries about the future. A friend, relative, minister, or family doctor can fulfill this role. He might consider seeking a therapist who can help him talk about, understand, and integrate his feelings. Whether a professional or a friend, a newly widowed man needs somebody who can be a caring listener. Feelings produced by the death of a spouse—or by divorce—if not allowed expression, disrupt people's lives. Anger or depression prevent a man from making the transition to a successful single again life.

If your wife died of a long, drawn-out disease such as cancer, accepting the fact of her death was one of the most difficult tasks imaginable. Yet, it allowed you to prepare and engage in anticipatory grieving. It was better for you and your dying spouse to deal with reality than keep up a false front and pretend everything was going to be all right. A dying person needs closeness and support to help her accept the tragic reality. Attempting to maintain the pretense that all is well and she will recover isolates her in an envelope of unreality, denying her the chance to express her true thoughts and feelings. By being dishonest with the dying spouse, however good his intentions, the survivor makes it harder on himself. Not only must he bear the strain of keeping up a pretense, but this makes it impossible to go through the anticipatory grieving process with the dying spouse. If this is avoided, when death occurs, he is unprepared for the devastating effects of the loss.

SEXUAL ISSUES

What happens sexually during the wife's illness? The husband is likely to experience normal sexual desires. Feeling the need for sex when his wife is terminally ill is not something a man should be ashamed of. Sexual desire is a basic and natural part of being alive. The question is how to integrate affectionate and sexual needs with the reality of the spouse's dying.

Sexual relations can continue as long as it is mutually comfortable. If the wife's illness makes it impossible or painful for her to engage in intercourse, the couple can continue affectionate and sensual touch, from caressing and massaging to use of manual or oral stimulation to orgasm. There is nothing "perverse" or offensive about sexual contact when the spouse is terminally ill. A primary need of dying people is not to be rejected, ignored, or denied. She wants to feel cared about, worthwhile, and loved. One of the chief ways of affirming someone's worth is through touching, of which sexuality is an important expression, although not the primary one.

In the latter stages of illness, sex may be unwanted or not possible. Masturbation can serve as an excellent sexual outlet. He should not feel childish or selfish for engaging in masturbation, it is a sensible way to satisfy his very human needs within the constraints of the situation. Another possibility is for the husband to seek a sexual affair. Some couples have an implicit understanding that it is all right for him to become sexually involved with another woman. Careful thought should be given, however, before proceeding. Since sexual relations often lead to feelings of emotional closeness, he might find a sexual liaison interferes with the closeness he wants with his spouse. Ultimately, it is a matter of weighing the alternatives—something each man must decide for himself according to his circumstances and value system.

Once the death of the spouse has occurred, the widower faces a different set of sexual issues. Although he has lost his wife, he has not lost his sexual capacity or desire. It is important the widower be aware his sexual feelings are normal. Sexuality is part of the life affirming process. He shouldn't be embarrassed or ashamed of sexual feelings. His sexual interest is positive, an indication of his will to survive and continue an active and fulfilling life.

He may go through a period of exploration and experimentation to determine the best way, given his present needs and feelings, of expressing himself sexually. Some men find sex is not important, but many more wish to find a way of integrating sexual activity into their lives. There are several options. For many widowers, masturbation is a helpful and enjoyable way to express sexuality. Masturbation is not harmful, at this or any other time. The widower should also be able, without feeling guilty, to think about and try a variety of sexual and life patterns until he finds one that suits his needs and values. He might seek a partner for marriage; he might want a stable partner for sex and companionship without marriage; or he might wish to have a variety of briefer, sexual friendships. Frequenting massage parlors or prostitutes may also be an alternative, although the need for intimacy and affection is less likely to be satisfied in this way.

A major issue widowers encounter is feeling they are being unfaithful to their dead wife. The standard folklore is "women grieve, men replace." The widower needs to realize it will not bring back his spouse if he deprives himself of emotional and sexual satisfaction; it will just make his life unhappy and difficult. He owes it to himself to gain as much happiness as possible after the death of the spouse—most wives who care for their husbands would not want it any other way. A sexual relationship can be an important source of satisfaction. The fact he has sex doesn't mean he didn't love his wife; it means he is a healthy male who chooses to continue his life despite his loss.

THE WIDOWER'S SYNDROME

When he does find a new partner, the widower might find he is out of practice sexually. Sex is a natural physiological response, but making love is a skill. Just as you do not play tennis or piano very well after several months or years away from it, when you begin sexual activity with a new partner you might feel awkward and need time to regain comfort and confidence. Anxiety, guilt, and other feelings intrude, causing erectile difficulty, early ejaculation, or ejaculatory inhibition. These difficulties are not unusual, and the man need not overreact or be discouraged. Through practice, he can regain sexual comfort and confidence. If the sexual problems continue for more than six months, he and his partner can consult a sex therapist.

As he forms a new emotional and sexual attachment, the widower should avoid making comparisons between his new partner and former wife. Experiences, both sexual and emotional, are likely to be very different from those with the spouse. Comparisons will not do anyone any good. Idealizing the deceased wife puts pressure on the new partner and causes her to feel discouraged and unloved. On the other hand, if the widower sees the new partner as superior, it leads to feelings of guilt. A healthier course is for the man to refrain from making comparisons and deal with the new relationship on its own merits.

CLOSING THOUGHTS

Each widowed or divorced man faces issues which are unique to his special circumstances. We have attempted to deal with some of the most important sexual issues. Being widowed or divorced is difficult, an experience that causes pain, anguish, depression, and self-doubt. No matter how rationally we deal with this, we cannot hope to escape entirely from its negative effects. However, by keeping in mind our basic worth as men and human beings, by remaining positive about ourselves and affirming our right to happiness and fulfillment, we can recover from the loss and reorganize our lives. By affirming our sexuality and expressing sexual feelings in a healthy way, we affirm ourselves as people. The single again man is aware he has a number of alternatives, he chooses what fits his situation and is in his best interest.

19
BEING GAY

Traditionally, books on sex treated homosexuality, if they dealt with it at all, as a problem to be changed. It was assumed homosexuality was abnormal, something had gone wrong in development, causing the man to prefer a type of sexual expression that was unnatural and perverted. Homosexuals were believed to be unhappy and desperately lonely. Homosexuality was thought of as a sickness, and, like any sickness, had an etiology (specific cause) and a cure. The trouble was no one was able to identify either the cause or the cure.

There has been a major change in attitudes and scientific knowledge about homosexuality in the past 20 years. In addition, there has been an active gay movement (much like the movements of other minority groups) to demand respect and equality. Prominent people have openly declared their homosexual orientation, and great numbers of others have "come out of the closet." Phrases such as "gay pride" and "gay is good" are commonplace. Findings by psychologists and other researchers challenge assumptions the straight world so smugly held about homosexuality. Research demonstrates homosexuality is not a disease. Homosexuality is a normal variant of human sexual expression, no less "natural" or "healthy" than other forms of sexuality.

The only sense in which homosexuality is "abnormal" is in the context of the values and beliefs held by people of a particular society. What is normal and desirable in one society may be abnormal or undesirable in another. Although homosexuality has existed in all times and all cultures, attitudes toward it have varied widely. In some instances it has been accepted as normal (as, for instance, in ancient Greece); in other instances it has been condemned as sinful, perverse, and punishable by death (as in fundamentalist Iran). But homosexuality has remained constant—nothing more nor less than a powerful emotional and sexual attraction for partners of the same sex. Whether this preference is considered an abomination or a personal right depends upon the values and attitudes of the people doing the judging.

In the United States, laws and attitudes toward homosexuality are in a stage of reevaluation. There are a bewildering number of misconceptions, superstitions, and glaringly myth-based notions, even among the most sophisticated strata of the population. With the growing strength of fundamentalist religious groups and fears raised by AIDS, there has been a backlash of prejudice. This chapter will attempt to dispel mistaken ideas, specifically with respect to male homosexuality, by exploring the subject in as factual and nonbiased a manner as possible.

DATA ABOUT HOMOSEXUALITY

One widely held, but erroneous, notion is that people must be either exclusively heterosexual or exclusively homosexual. Alfred Kinsey introduced the concept that homosexuality and heterosexuality can be envisioned as falling along a continuum, rather than an either-or dichotomy. The sex histories of many men revealed both heterosexual and homosexual feelings and experiences. For example, an adolescent might have homosexual experiences, but as an adult be emotionally and sexually committed to women. Another man, who has most of his sexual relationships with males, occasionally becomes sexually involved with a woman.

Approximately 75 percent of men have had at least one fantasy, thought, or feeling about another male that caused them to become aroused, usually occurring during adolescence or early adulthood. It is estimated one out of four men has at least one homosexual experience leading to orgasm sometime in his life, usually in adolescence or early adulthood. One in ten has been sexual with men for at least a year in his life. About 3-6 percent of males have a homosexual orientation.[16] These facts are particularly important for heterosexual men who mistakenly believe their sexual orientation must be pure and untainted. They fear homosexual thoughts or same sex experiences make them "latent homosexuals." The term *latent homosexuality* is neither accurate nor useful. It serves to make men afraid and to reinforce homophobic feelings. This rampant homophobia is the reason that members of the gay community are more likely to be victims of violent physical attacks than almost any other minority in the U.S. Males are so afraid of homosexual thoughts, feelings, fantasies, and/or experiences that they overreact by being angry or belittling toward gay men.

HOMOSEXUALITY IS NOT A MENTAL ILLNESS

Another common misconception is that homosexuality is a form of mental illness. Many people regard it as common sense that anyone who prefers partners of the same sex to partners of the opposite sex must be "sick." Books and articles written by psychiatrists reinforce this point of view. But these writings are based on clinical theory rather than scientific evidence, with the case studies drawn from the psychiatrist's patients—clearly a biased sample.

There is a good deal of scientific evidence to indicate homosexuality does not involve more pathology than heterosexuality. Family pressures and the societal and economic discrimination homosexuals have to deal with add considerable stress to their lives. In acknowledgment of such evidence and in response to pressure from the gay community, both the American Psychological Association and the American Psychiatric Association have adopted as their official position that homosexuality is not deviant behavior and is within the normal range of sexual expression. This view is accepted by the great majority of sex researchers and sex educators, including Masters and Johnson and the Kinsey Institute. For homosexual men, being gay is their optimal identity. The issue is how to live their lives psychologically, relationally, sexually, professionally, and in terms of health in the most fulfilling manner.

Homosexuality is best understood as an emotional and sexual commitment to the same sex, not as an illness or social problem. As long as homosexuality (or any form of sexual activity) is freely agreed upon by both partners, performed in private, not coercive, not compulsive, does not cause physical injury, does not involve children, and is not used to inflict guilt or punishment on oneself or one's partner, it is within the range of normal sexual behavior. This is not to say homosexuality is in any way better than heterosexuality or that everyone should try it. Homosexuality needs to be accepted as valid for the 3-6 percent of men who are gay.

PREJUDICE AGAINST GAYS

People believe homosexual men can be identified by certain physical characteristics or peculiarities of dress and behavior. People feel their ability to identify homosexuals shows perceptiveness or sophistication, but in reality it is a sign of prejudice similar to that of the anti-Semite who is convinced he can "always spot a Jew." Actually, most gays cannot be identified by outward signs. Nor is it true that gays are found exclusively in certain occupations such as interior decorating or hairdressing. There are gays in every field of endeavor, including stevedores, business executives, athletes, machinists, doctors, truck drivers, ministers and college professors. Some gays, of course, do dress and act in a flamboyantly effeminate manner, but they are in the minority. This is a source of disagreement in the gay community, some applauding the public display of gayness, others objecting to those who flaunt their homosexuality.

Despite the recent liberalization of attitudes, society continues to be ambivalent or hostile. Although the military has recently adopted a "don't ask, don't tell" policy, there is significant discrimination against homosexuals. In spite of a movement among the clergy to incorporate gays into the religious community, the Roman Catholic Church and fundamentalist Protestant churches continues to regard homosexuality as a perversion. Moreover, the attitude of most people toward homosexuality is poor, ranging from tolerance to disgust. What are the reasons for this widespread and persistent antagonism?

It has to do with the mistaken belief that homosexuality is on the upswing and unless kept down by force it will threaten the integrity of the family and the structure of society. There is no basis for this fear. Research indicates there has been no change in the percentage of men who have a homosexual orientation. Homosexuality has become more visible because more individuals have openly declared themselves rather than live a hidden or double life. Contrary to the fears of "family values" advocates, homosexuality does not pose a threat to the family. The great majority of males have been and will continue to be heterosexual; they will marry and produce more than enough children to ensure the perpetuation of society. In truth, "hate is not a family value."

AIDS is the newest reason to excuse antihomosexual prejudices. Although AIDS is a very serious public health problem and of major concern to gay men, it is neither a homosexual nor a heterosexual disease, but a disease which is sexually spread primarily by men.

Another reason people fear homosexuality is they are convinced homosexuals are child molesters. The man who goes about seducing young boys is a figure of fear for anxious parents. In truth, the majority of child sex abusers prey on young girls. Although there is a genuine problem of sexual abuse of male children, these men are pedophiles—men attracted to children—not homosexuals.

A related, but more subtle fear, is increased acceptance of homosexuality will cause the male role to become ambiguous and make it more likely young boys will become homosexual. Many people are particularly opposed to gays as teachers because they fear the teacher would steer a boy toward homosexuality at the point in his life when he is most impressionable and his sexual identity is in the process of formation. However, research argues these concerns, too, are largely groundless. Increased awareness and acceptance does not lead to increased homosexuality.

Perhaps the most significant reason heterosexual men are hostile to gays has to do with an apprehension that their heterosexual orientation is ambiguous or tenuous. Heterosexual men are afraid of being "contaminated" by contact with homosexuals, which is the basis for homophobia. The heterosexual feels threatened because he fears there is a homosexual part of him the gay man might recognize and make a play for. This is responsible for the overreaction of straight men to sexual overtures by gays. The heterosexual feels he has to protect his manhood by reacting rudely, threateningly, or even by beating up the gay male. Straight males harass gay men on the street to show how "macho" they are. A man who is secure with his heterosexual orientation feels no need to react this way. He recognizes the invitation for what it is—a mistake, a misdirected attempt to attract a sexual partner—and responds by ignoring it or assertively saying he is not interested.

Heterosexuals are particularly threatened because of the subtle indoctrination men in our society receive against physical contact between males. We learn early that male contact should be strictly limited (to competitive sports, a slap on the back, a handshake). Even in father-son relationships, touching, roughhousing, and hugging comes to a halt as the boy grows older. Supposedly this restraint is to maintain the social ideal of being "male." In contrast, women are freer to express themselves physically and emotionally. The demonstration of affection between women is accepted and does not arouse fears it will promote lesbianism or undermine female identity. The person who loses to this irrational fear is the heterosexual man who would benefit from an affectionate hug with his best friend or child.

CAUSES OF HOMOSEXUALITY

Although many theories have been posited to explain why people are homosexual, the question remains unanswered. The traditional question is "What went wrong to cause homosexuality?" This is biased and unscientific, since it assumes homosexuality involves a psychological or physical malfunction. A popular psychiatric theory suggests homosexuals are the products of families in which there is a dominant and seductive mother and a passive or absent father. Although the backgrounds of some conform to this pattern, it is not true for the majority of gay men. The leading theory is homosexuality has a physiological basis, either genetic or a fetal hormone mechanism that predisposes homosexuality. If this were true, it would make biases against homosexuals less acceptable since the person has no control over sexual orientation.

Another approach is to view sexual orientation, whether homosexual or heterosexual, as a complex phenomenon influenced by many interconnected factors—genetics, hormones, child-rearing practices, peer interactions, sex education (or lack thereof), body image, history of comfort and attraction, relationships between men and women, and early sexual experiences.

It is possible that a series of "pleasure events" in the presence of a member of the same sex culminate in a strong attraction for men—a process analogous to what we hypothesize happens in the development of heterosexuality. Early orgasmic experiences might be particularly important. Sexual fantasies used during masturbation, especially if focused on one theme (sexual attraction to blue-eyed, blond men in their twenties or being passive in anal intercourse), could have a strong reinforcing effect on sexual orientation.

Perhaps the most compelling explanation is sexual orientation is a multicausal, multidimensional phenomena with many individual differences and determinants. Regardless of what causes homosexuality, the most sensible and least prejudicial way of understanding sexual orientation is as a commitment to a life which is in accordance with the man's emotional and sexual needs. Whether a person commits to homosexuality, heterosexuality, or bisexuality, this ought to be respected by others, regardless of whether they share or approve of that orientation. It may be some time before such acceptance is reached in our society, but it is sure to bring greater happiness and fulfillment than possible under prejudiced, repressive attitudes.

WHAT GAY MEN DO SEXUALLY

A great many misconceptions center around the methods used by gays to obtain sexual pleasure. People assume the sexual practices of gays include strange rituals with "kinky" and perverse acts. This exemplifies the tendency of people to impute strange behavior to a group of which they have little knowledge. Although some gays do practice "exotic" sexual behavior, the percentage is no greater than among heterosexuals. The sexual techniques used by gay couples are identical to those used by heterosexuals—which underscores the absurdity of identifying any sexual technique as homosexual. A homosexual interaction is defined by the fact that two same-sex people are involved, not by the nature of the sex act. For example, oral sex is heterosexual if opposite-sex partners are involved and homosexual if same-sex partners are involved.

Fellatio is a form of sexual behavior commonly enjoyed by gays. Fellatio might be mutual ("69" position), or experienced by one partner at a time. It might be used as an arousal technique or carried to orgasm. Manual stimulation as a pleasuring technique or to orgasm is common. Gays use self-stimulation with a partner present more than heterosexual men. They are more likely to use rubbing stimulation and interfemoral intercourse (thrusting the penis between the partner's thighs).

Anal intercourse is the most controversial sexual technique. Contrary to popular thinking, anal intercourse is not the primary sexual act for gay men. Being passive in anal intercourse is the highest risk behavior for HIV/AIDS. Some couples take turns being the active (insertive) partner, while others have a strong preference for either the active or passive role. Interestingly, the preference for being passive is five times more common. Safer sex guidelines emphasize the crucial importance of using a condom each time. In Barry's clinical work with men who are passive in anal intercourse, he encourages both partners be tested for HIV. If one partner is HIV positive, anal intercourse, even with a condom, is strongly discouraged.

It is important to note that all of these sexual activities (including anal intercourse) are engaged in by heterosexual as well as homosexual couples. The only activity exclusive to heterosexuals is penis-vagina intercourse. Gays use sexual techniques with as much variation and imagination (or lack of it) as do heterosexuals. Kissing, caressing, and other pleasuring activities that are part of heterosexual encounters are commonly incorporated into gay lovemaking as well.

Some sexual encounters—such as anonymous sex in men's bathrooms or at a gay bar—are devoid of affection and emotion. But then so are most encounters between heterosexual men and prostitutes or one-night stands at bars. These sexual experiences do not promote physical or mental health, and have become less frequent with fears of HIV/AIDS. Condoms should be used or there should be no exchange of semen.

Men who limit their homosexual encounters to brief, impersonal meetings are attempting to maintain a heterosexual facade and satisfy their preference for male sexual contact on the sly. If the man is married, this puts both himself and his spouse at risk. The anonymity and lack of warmth may be blamed partially on the repressive intolerance of heterosexual society and partially on the cultural myth that erotic sex is high risk, intense, and nonintimate.

Gays need and seek out closeness and intimacy. Each man may have sexual preferences, but should not be inflexible, engaging only in stereotypical, rigid sexual behavior. Like his heterosexual counterpart, he feels the need for sexual spontaneity, variety and emotional satisfaction.

GAY LIFESTYLES

Lifestyles among gays are diverse—a fact that runs counter to the myth that gays are obsessed with making sexual contacts to the exclusion of other life experiences. They succeed in integrating homosexuality into their lives, engage in productive occupations, have a range of social and cultural interests, and establish satisfying friendships, as well as a romantic and sexual union with a lover. Because of the stigma attached to homosexuality, many gays express their sexual orientation clandestinely, admitting they are homosexual only to other gays, while representing themselves as straight to the rest of the world. They lead two separate lives, maintaining separate identities. The psychological stress is wearing. They are not yet able or willing to join gays who are open, vocal, and assertive in affirming their sexual orientation, who proclaim homosexuality is not a second-rate human condition and that being gay need not involve shame, guilt, or an apologetic attitude.

Like any minority group, gays place a high value on social institutions that allow them to enjoy the company of others who share their preferences and problems. Hence, the continuing popularity of gay bars. The gay bar serves the same purpose for homosexuals as the singles bar serves for heterosexuals. Not all gay men enjoy the bar scene; some, in fact, avoid bars, preferring activities such as dinner parties, social action groups, or team sports. "Cruising" (seeking out sexual contacts) involves walking or driving in areas where there is a heavy concentration of men seeking sexual liaisons. Cruising—whether it occurs in a bar, party, class, or at an intersection—involves a subtle and complex system of nonverbal cues. In some areas, male prostitution ("hustling") occurs.

Sexual relationships between gay men are less permanent than heterosexual relationships or relationships between lesbians. To a certain extent, this impermanence can be attributed to the corrosive effect of society's negative attitude toward gay attachments. Long-term relationships between heterosexual couples are encouraged in a multitude of ways by society (including legal, financial, and property advantages), particularly when formalized by marriage and involving children. Female homosexuality, while not approved by society, arouses less hostility. Women are traditionally allowed to be more physically expressive; unmarried women can comfortably live together as roommates. A lesbian couple can maintain a relationship without attracting as much attention as a gay couple.

Nevertheless, many gays establish relationships that last five, ten, twenty years, a lifetime. Some gay couples have, in fact, sought to legitimize their relationships as formal marriages, insisting that to deny them the same rights and advantages accorded heterosexual couples constitutes blatant discrimination. There is growing support for permanent, monogamous gay relationships.

Gays have organized in other ways. The Gay Activist Alliance, along with other advocacy groups, is working for an end to discrimination in hiring practices, living arrangements, and other societal institutions. Gay religious groups are attempting to bring about the acceptance of homosexuality within the religious establishment. There are gay community churches, "Dignity" groups, masses for gay Episcopalians, temples for gay Jews. These organizations underscore the fact that gays are human beings whose sexual orientation and lifestyle is legitimate and should in no way preclude them from enjoying the same freedom and privileges accorded to others. "Problem-centered" groups and services such as "gay Alcoholics Anonymous," gay switchboards, and gay clinics have been established to deal with specific difficulties. The gay community has established a strong network of support groups and services for PWA's (people with AIDS). Fighting the HIV/AIDS epidemic by enlisting community support has had a positive effect on many gay men and the gay community.

DECISION MAKING ABOUT SEXUAL ORIENTATION

As we observed earlier, sexual orientation falls along a continuum, with some men experiencing arousal in both homosexual and heterosexual interactions. Why shouldn't they be able to express themselves with men and women? Most men find it quite difficult to function as bisexuals. Straddling both worlds places serious social and psychological stresses on the individual which are difficult to sustain. The number of men who are genuinely bisexual, with equal emotional and sexual attraction to both men and women, is very small.

A commitment to a sexual identity (orientation) ultimately rests with the individual based on what he feels would lead to the greatest pleasure, fulfillment, and happiness. His decision should not be based on what others want for him—whether parents, a wife, religion, an employer, or society at large. People who are closest believe they know what is best for him, but their emotional involvement makes it difficult to provide unbiased and nonjudgmental advice. It is the individual himself who must live with the decision, so it is he who must assume responsibility for it.

Nor is it advisable to procrastinate when making a commitment regarding sexual orientation. Difficult as life may be for gays in certain instances, there are few things more painful for a man than to go through the motions of heterosexual existence while fighting against the awareness that his true emotional and sexual needs would be fulfilled with a man. A common mistake is to marry as an attempt to avoid the issue. These marriages turn out to be shams where the man is leading a double life. One of the most difficult situations is the man who, fearing to confront his homosexual orientation, chooses to deny his sexual needs altogether and makes no sexual contacts with people of either sex. He condemns himself to living a shadow existence.

We are sexual beings whether we admit it or not, with a right to emotional and sexual satisfaction. To deny this is to shut off one of the major sources of happiness in life—but that, too, is

an individual decision. For a man making the commitment to a
sexual orientation, therapy can be invaluable. A therapist, if he
is competent and well-trained, will not attempt to force a particular decision. The therapist's role is to help the man discover
what his real needs are and assist in planning a course of action
designed to realize them. This professional may be a psychologist, minister, clinical social worker, psychiatrist, or a counselor
at a gay counseling service. His effectiveness will depend less
on professional credentials than on his commitment to helping
the man reach a personally satisfying decision. Barry has seen a
number of men in therapy seeking help in committing to a sexual
orientation. Barry's guiding principle is the needs and desires of
the person come first. A solution to the issue (or any sexual
problem) imposed externally is no solution at all.

Tom

Tom was a nineteen-year-old college student who had been
sexually active with men since he was thirteen. The summer
before, Tom's parents found out about his homosexual activities
and insisted he seek therapy. Tom presented as a reluctant client,
making it clear he was coming to a therapist under duress and
expected Barry to share his parents' disapproving attitude.
Barry's first task was to make clear he viewed homosexuality as
a valid sexual identity and it was not his intention to force
change.

We agreed to spend three sessions reviewing Tom's sexual
development and preferences and then determine a plan of action. In a careful assessment of Tom's attitudes, behavior, emotions, attraction, and sexual functioning, it was clear his
commitment was to men. His sexual experiences, masturbatory
fantasies, and emotional and sexual preferences pointed toward
an overwhelming attraction to men. We focused on how to discuss his homosexual identity with his parents in a way they could
accept without blaming themselves for Tom being gay. It was
unrealistic to expect them to be enthusiastic about his commitment. Acceptance was the most Tom could hope for. This turned
out to be the right approach; Tom's parents eventually became
reconciled to his homosexual identity, which contributed greatly
toward relieving tension in the family. The parents joined P-Flag,

a self-help group for parents of gay people. This allowed Tom to focus on his crucial issues—how to be successful as a gay person psychologically, sexually, and emotionally. The commitment to leading a successful and satisfying life is an integral part of accepting one's homosexuality. For Tom, being gay was optimal. Tom's challenge was to organize his life as a gay man to enhance psychological and sexual well-being.

George
Another client, George, was a twenty-one-year-old who felt very confused and ambivalent about his sexual orientation. It was a constant source of anxiety and obsession. Since the age of fourteen, he felt admiration and attraction for athletic, virile men. Convinced he had a small penis, George was aroused by the thought of men with large organs. Although George masturbated frequently to a variety of homosexual, heterosexual, bisexual, and group sexual fantasies, his sexual experiences were limited. He'd had two successful homosexual experiences in which he was fellated to orgasm, and one unsuccessful heterosexual intercourse in which he ejaculated before he could insert his penis into the woman's vagina.

George sought therapy to discuss his confused sexual feelings. Ultimately, the decision about sexual orientation is the man's responsibility. A therapist cannot tell you whether you're straight or gay. After five sessions in which we explored his sexual experiences, feelings, values, and fantasies, George decided the best fit for him was a commitment to a heterosexual orientation. Therapy focused on a systematic program to increase heterosexual skills and arousal and decrease homosexual obsessions. This process proved successful. George was able to experience both sexual arousal and emotional intimacy with women in a way he could not with males.

A RATIONAL VIEW OF HOMOSEXUALITY
For the sake of homosexuals and heterosexuals alike, it would be best if society could adopt the principle that serves as a guide for responsible therapists: sexual orientation is a matter the individual himself must be free to decide in his best interest. Those

committing to a homosexual identitiy should be given as much respect as those who are heterosexual. Homosexuality should be accepted as a truly alternative way of life, not a second-class one. A gay person is above all a human being and society should emphasize the positive aspects of his humanness rather than stigmatize him with the label of deviant or abnormal. Contrary to folk myths, there is such a thing as a successful gay person. In his professional work, Barry has seen quite a few well-functioning and some optimally functioning gay men. Whether we will meet more in the future depends at least in part on the attitude straights adopt. The most important element, however, is the self-acceptance of the gay person and his commitment to be successful in his emotional and sexual life.

20
MEN AND SEXUAL TRAUMA

When people discuss sexual trauma, they identify women as victims and men as perpetrators. Men can't be victims of sexual trauma—it happens only to women. This myth is powerful, painful, and stigmatizing for males who have experienced abusive and/or traumatic sexual incidents.

Sexual trauma is a complex, sensitive, and controversial area that involves men in three ways. The first is males as victims of sexual incidents, especially child sexual abuse and incest. Second, males as perpetrators of sexual incidents, especially rape, child sexual abuse, incest, exhibitionism, voyeurism, and sexual harassment. Third, the male as a helper in the healing process when his wife, partner, son, or daughter has been sexually traumatized. These are separate issues, although some men experience two or all three of these problems.

Dealing with sexual trauma cannot be achieved through reading a book, attending a lecture, watching a TV program, or listening to a talk show. This increases awareness and understanding, but is not sufficient. Resolving sexual trauma is an issue for professional therapy. What we hope to do in this chapter is increase awareness and suggest guidelines for addressing the issues.

THE MALE WHO IS SEXUALLY TRAUMATIZED

Let us begin with the male as a victim of sexual trauma. An upsetting statistic is that by age 16, approximately one in seven male children will have a significant sexual interaction with an adult.[17] If you define negative sexual experiences broadly—to include contracting a sexually transmitted disease, being sexually humiliated, causing an unwanted pregnancy, guilt over masturbation, having a sexual dysfunction, trapped in a compulsive sexual pattern, being sexually rejected—in addition to the major trauma of child sexual abuse, incest, and rape (by a man), you are confronted with a disturbing realization. Negative, confusing, abusive, or traumatic sexual experiences are an almost universal phenomena for men (as well as women). Over 90 percent of men can identify at least one sexual incident (whether in childhood, adolescence, or adulthood) that caused negative feelings, guilt, confusion, and/or trauma.

The stigma and sense of victimization is more psychologically traumatic than the sexual incident itself. For example, a nine-year-old boy who is sexually abused by a neighbor or boy scout leader treats this as a shameful secret, telling no one. The boy feels shamed by the incident, as if he did something wrong or caused the abuse. He has to deal with a triple stigma: 1) abuse is supposed to happen to girls, not boys, 2) because it's a same sex incident, he fears the stigma of homosexuality, 3) males are supposed to be strong and streetwise, so he must be weak or deficient. Even if he tells someone, there is a tendency among adults to not believe the boy's accusations and/or to be angry at him. Our culture "blames the victim." This tendency is at its worst in incidents of sexual abuse of boys. It is better to reveal abuse than keep the incident a secret, feelings of shame and guilt multiply with secrecy. A therapeutic adage is "you're only as sick as your secrets."

When the incident is disclosed, the boy's needs are seldom listened to or met. The child wants to understand the abusive incident, not feel blamed for it, and he wants the abuse to stop. Usually he wants to continue a relationship with the man, as long as it's nonabusive. Instead, the result of disclosure is more confusion, anxiety, depression, and stigma. When the incident is dealt with badly by parents, friends, police, or the school system it increases confusion and guilt. He blames himself for not having been stronger and/or maintaining control. The abuse has stopped, but the guilt and stigma remain, and often are stronger.

The child who keeps the incident secret and tries to deny it happened is likely to feel depressed. The secret becomes powerful and controlling of his personal and sexual self-esteem. The child blames himself, feeling like a victim with a shameful secret.

The most maladaptive pattern is the boy who deals with the sexual abuse by the "super macho" strategy of becoming a perpetrator and sexually abusing other children. On reviewing the history of pedophiles, almost half were sexually abused as children. So the pattern of abuse continues, claiming more victims. There is no justification for sexually abusing children; that is a destructive way to rebuild masculine control.

The central issue for an adult is whether the man sees himself as a "survivor" or a "victim." Viewing himself as a victim and allowing the trauma to control his life is a more severe form of victimization than the original abuse or how it was dealt with at the time. It is crucial for him to learn to be a sexual survivor. This means he accepts the sexual incidents, acknowledges he coped as well as he could and did survive, doesn't blame himself but places the responsibility where it belongs—on the perpetrator, learns from the abuse, feels responsible for himself and his sexuality, is committed to living well sexually and psychologically, and sees himself as a proud survivor, not a passive victim. He is committed to not perpetuate the cycle of abuse. He is not abusive to either children or adult women.

The reality of sexual trauma cannot be denied or minimized. Neither should it control self-esteem or sexuality. The man needs support from friends, family, community, and professionals to cope with the trauma. He is an active survivor rather than a passive victim. The most helpful cognition is "living well is the best revenge." The man who feels responsible for his sexuality, has integrated past abuse into his self-esteem, is committed to sexual expression which is voluntary, mutual, and pleasure-oriented, and who can experience desire, arousal, orgasm, and satisfaction in an intimate relationship, takes pride and satisfaction in being a survivor.

MEN AS PERPETRATORS OF SEXUAL TRAUMA

Who perpetrates sexual trauma? Men. In over 90 percent of sexual trauma (with female or male victims) the perpetrator is a male. Why is it that child sexual abuse, incest, rape, exhibitionism, voyeurism, sexual harassment and obscene phone calls are done by males? Abuse is multicausal, but there are two major factors. First, is our old nemesis the double standard. Taken to its illogical extreme, it says the man has a right to be sexual with any woman, any time, and in any situation. If there's not an available and willing adult female, he may feel he has a right to force or coerce an adolescent, child, or even senior citizen. This is the rationale behind acquaintance rape. The destructive belief is "an erect penis has no conscience." This is the mistaken assumption behind abusive male sexual behavior. The second factor is that between 2-5 percent of males have a paraphiliac arousal pattern. This means sexual arousal to someone or something which is not an appropriate arousal source.

There are "benign" paraphilias, which means the arousal pattern does not harm others. Examples include fetishes (to shoes, rubber, hair, etc), bondage and discipline, cross-dressing, or cybersex. The "noxious" paraphilias include exhibitionism (flashers), voyeurism (Peeping Toms), pedophiles (child molesters), frotteurs (rubbing his penis against a woman, especially on buses and subways), and obscene phone callers. A noxious paraphilia means the sexual behavior causes at least discomfort and often trauma for the victim. Noxious paraphilias are illegal acts, and the man is criminally liable.

There is scientific controversy about whether a genetic predisposition, a neurological impairment, or inappropriate learning causes a paraphilia. What is clear is males develop this sexual compulsion before adolescence. It is reinforced by obsessive paraphiliac masturbatory fantasies which become more controlling and compelling over time. A paraphilia is a compulsive, addictive behavior which limits the man's ability to enjoy sexuality to a very narrow range of stimuli. In the case of noxious paraphilias, it results in psychological trauma to others, even though this is not the man's intent.

FETISHES

A man with a fetish arousal pattern has a powerful compulsive sexual arousal to a specific stimulus, but only mild (or absent) arousal to partner eroticism and intercourse. For example, he feels overwhelming arousal to an inanimate object like leather or panty hose, but minimal arousal to the woman's touch. Many men with fetish arousal are able to function sexually early in a relationship, but as the relationship continues their desire and arousal dissipates. The fetish material or fantasy serves as a wall which blocks emotional and sexual connection. The majority of males use fantasy during partner sex, which serves as a bridge to arousal with the partner—fantasy facilitates involvement. Fetish fantasy or material controls the man's arousal. When he is fantasizing about panty hose it serves to block out the partner so he can focus on the real source of his arousal (the fetish). Another example is the man who is a transvestite (cross-dresser). He claims he dresses in a bra because it allows him to have greater sexual pleasure with his wife. The truth is he *needs* the cross-dressing to *enable* him to function sexually. The three factors which differentiate a fetish from the normal variations of sexual arousal are the elements of *controlling* sexual arousal, *narrowness* of the stimulus and serving to *wall off* the man rather than be a bridge for involvement and arousal.

Sexuality is an intimate sharing of pleasure. A paraphilia is best understood as an intimacy disorder, reducing emotional and sexual involvement.

NOXIOUS PARAPHILIAS

These refer to compulsive sexual arousal patterns which have a negative effect on others as well as putting the man in legal jeopardy—exhibitionism, voyeurism, frotteurism, obscene phone calls. The most negative is pedophilia (child sexual abuse). Although the sexual behavior is harmful to others as well as self-destructive, the great majority of males with noxious paraphilias are decent people. However, their sexuality is controlled by a compulsive, harmful sexual pattern. This does not condone the sexual acting out; it must be confronted and stopped.

The pattern is the exhibitionist feels guilty about his deviant behavior, and it becomes the controlling secret of his life. He will not seek treatment until the sexual behavior is discovered by someone or he is arrested. In fact, exhibitionism is the sexual crime most likely to result in arrest. The exhibitionist has done this for years and has exposed himself to hundreds, perhaps thousands, of victims (usually girls or young women). The exhibitionist engages in cognitive distortions (self-deluding thoughts, such as he is providing sex education by exhibiting himself or the woman's look reflects how impressed she is by his erection). He needs to confront the reality of his sexual behavior—it is abusive, illegal, and harmful. There is no emotional, sexual, or legal justification for exhibitionistic behavior. There needs to be a commitment to totally abstain from exhibitionism (or other harmful sexual compulsions) and to therapy (often in addition to self-help sex addiction groups). The techniques to change deviant arousal involve aversive procedures (covert sensitization and shame aversion) and/or medication to reduce obsessive sexual fantasy and desire. Both for legal reasons and the harm this behavior causes others, the only viable goal is total abstinence.

PEDOPHILIA

Males whose noxious paraphilia involves sexual arousal to children under age 14 are called pedophiles (those who are sexually aroused by adolescents from 14 to 17 are called hebrophiles). The majority offend against female children, although a significant number offend against male children. This is the most negative and harmful paraphilia. The great majority of pedophiles do not use physical violence, do not engage in intercourse, nor do they want to harm the child. They feel inadequate in adult sexual relationships, but feel accepted, comfortable, and sexually aroused with children. About half the interactions with female children involve "hands-off" abuse—looking at, exhibiting himself, or verbal sexual harassment. "Hands-on" abuse involves fondling the child's breasts, vulva or anal area; having the child touch the man's penis; giving or receiving oral sex or other erotic contact. Sexual abuse of boys usually involves "hands-on" contact and is orgasm focused. The pedophile minimizes or rationalizes his sexual acting-out, denying it has a negative impact on the child. In fact, the issue is how much trauma it causes. Violent interactions (about 15 percent) are very traumatic. Interactions which are physically intrusive and orgasm focused (oral, anal, or vaginal sex) are also highly traumatic. Sexual abuse involving people the child knows and trusts (relatives, neighbors, teachers, ministers) are more traumatic than with strangers because a trust bond is broken. Repeated incidents of abuse where the child feels pressure to keep the secret are more traumatic than a single episode which is revealed and dealt with.

DEALING WITH INCEST

Incest is shrouded in blame and secrecy with the mistaken belief that incest occurs only in the most pathological families. Incest is abusive and harmful both psychologically and sexually. The most frequent forms of incestuous behavior involve cousins, in-laws, uncles, and siblings. The sexual interaction usually does not include intercourse, but does involve viewing, fondling, manual or oral stimulation. Most incest involves female children, but male children are sexually abused by uncles, brothers, in-laws, stepfathers, and fathers. The relationship which has the most negative impact is between a father and son or daughter.

There are many causes of incest and many forms of incestuous activity. The man will try to rationalize by saying ''it only happens when he's drinking,'' ''the child is seductive and enjoys it,'' ''his wife is nonsexual and it's better than an affair,'' ''the boy had an orgasm so how could it be abuse,'' ''it's not really sex because it didn't involve intercourse.'' These are rationalizations, meant to excuse or minimize. The truth is the man engages in incest to meet his selfish emotional and sexual needs at the expense of the child. Legally, psychologically, and sexually incest is a destructive behavior which has to be confronted and stopped.

Treatment involves the whole family, not just the man. What allows incest to continue is the secrecy. Once the secret is revealed, it is crucial that lines of communication remain open so the perpetrator and family members know incest will not be tolerated. Treatment requires a focus on the man individually, on couple therapy, and family therapy. Whether incest was provoked by the man's alcoholism, his pedophilia, personal or sexual inadequacy, the problem has to be dealt with so he cannot repeat incestuous behavior. If the marriage and family is to remain intact, the husband-wife bond of respect, trust, and intimacy needs to be restored. Incest does not occur in families where there is a functional husband-wife bond. Through family therapy, the mother's role as a positive factor in the family needs to be rebuilt. Often, the mother has been impaired either physically or psychologically and taken a passive role in the family. She needs to rebuild her self-esteem and relationship with the children so that, if another incident occurs, the child will turn to her for protection and she will be strong enough to demand that the perpetrator leave the house. The child has to be confident he is safe and will not be sexually revictimized. Children need to learn the healthy role of sexuality in life, and reestablish appropriate parent-child bonds. One component of therapy is a formal apology session where the perpetrator (whether father, brother, step-sibling) takes responsibility for the incest, apologizes, and commits to not repeating the destructive behavior. The mother apologizes for not being there to support and protect the children, and commits to being a strong, active force in the family. The child (children) agree in accepting the apology they will not use incest as a weapon to get their way in the family. Incest is no longer the controlling factor in the family or in the children's self-esteem. This is true whether the family remains intact or the perpetrator leaves the family.

Incest is very serious and destructive. It is an example of the man's inappropriate sexual desire causing harm to his children, himself, and the entire family. Incest cannot remain a shameful family secret, but needs to be confronted, dealt with, and stopped.

RAPE

Rape is the double standard taken to its most illogical extreme. Rape is the use of physical force and/or coercion (verbal or threat) to force the woman to engage in sex. Most states define rape as penis-vagina intercourse, but any forced sexual act is rape, which includes oral sex, anal intercourse, or manual sex. Men have justified rape by saying the woman led him on, she was asking for it, she could have stopped by closing her legs or fighting back. These are weak rationalizations to avoid facing his responsibility and the reality he's committed a violent crime. You cannot "blame the victim." Rape is the man's responsibility, period. No matter what she wore, how much she drank, what his friends said, or how sexually involved she was earlier in the evening, if the woman says "No," and the man forces a sexual act against her will, it's rape.

A concept used in rape prevention training which we strongly disagree with is "all men are potential rapists." This builds a paranoia between men and women, and perpetuates the double standard view of sexuality. Men who view women as people, not objects, will not rape. The more sexuality is understood as a voluntary, pleasurable sharing between equal, respectful partners, the less the likelihood of rape. Men, as well as women, individuals as well as the culture (including the legal system) need to adopt a strong, unequivocal stance against forced or coercive sex.

Each year there are over 100,000 rapes reported to the police. Only one in five rapes is reported. Rape is a crime which is increasing in frequency. Sometime in their lives one in four women will be a rape or attempted rape victim. Although the most publicized type of rape is perpetrated by a stranger with a weapon, the most common type is "acquaintance rape"—a date, someone she knows from work, a friend of a friend, or someone she met in a bar or at a dance.

Rape is an act of violence, not just a sexual act. However, being raped is different from being mugged. The combination of violence and sexuality makes rape a particularly traumatic experience. Two-thirds of women report psychological distress three months after the rape. Rape is not a minor life experience to shrug off. Rape not only affects the woman, but significant people in her life including family, friends, a boyfriend or spouse. These people are co-victims. They feel the stress and are unsure how to react to her or to communicate how they feel.

There are a number of theories of why men rape and categories of rapists. Many rapists are married or have regular sex partners which belies the excuse that the man needs a sexual outlet. Males rape because they feel it is their right to dominate and humiliate the woman. They believe when it comes to sex the man has a right to what he can get away with. The incidence of rape will continue to grow unless men, individually and as a group, forcefully state it is wrong, will not be tolerated, and will be punished.

THE MALE AS A PARTNER IN HEALING

When a man learns his wife has been raped, his son has been sexually abused by a youth leader, or his daughter was exhibited to by a brother-in-law, his first reaction is anger and the desire to harm the perpetrator. The problem is you are reacting to your angry needs instead of the needs of your child or spouse. The macho role of being angry and violent is not in the best interest of your spouse, children, or the healing process.

When you learn your child has been sexually abused, focus on helping the child become a survivor rather than a victim. Begin by helping him (or her) accept the complex reality of the sexual abuse, with all the attendant thoughts and feelings (positive and negative, rational and irrational). Second, listen to him in a caring way—find out what he is feeling, what happened, and what help he wants from you. Third, help him understand the responsibility for the abuse lies with the perpetrator, not the child. The child need not blame himself nor feel guilty. Fourth, the child deserves the understanding, support, and help of family, friends, school, community, counselors and police. Fifth, this traumatic event can be an opportunity to provide positive sexuality education. Last, and most important, the child is helped to acknowledge that he coped and survived. His self-esteem is of a survivor and winner, not a victim and loser. A favorite adage is "living well is the best revenge." The survivor can emerge from the abuse as a stronger, more aware child who will make sexuality a positive part of his growing up and adulthood.

What if your spouse (or dating partner) has been raped? How can you be an active participant in the healing process? The rape of a spouse or partner is a difficult experience for a man. He feels a range of emotions from anger and rage to disgust and helplessness. Although irrational, it is easier for him to be supportive if it was a stranger rape and/or there was violence. In a nonviolent (i.e., no weapons or bruises) acquaintance rape, the male easily falls into the trap of blaming the woman and taking his anger out on her. He questions her judgment and calls her stupid for getting into the vulnerable situation. By blaming his partner he is doubly victimizing her and harming their relationship. She needs acceptance and support, not your criticisms and put-downs.

What she needs is for you to listen in a respectful, caring

manner. Her feelings and needs come first in dealing with this crisis. In a rape, the perpetrator's needs are met at the woman's expense, sex is forced or coerced, her physical and emotional boundaries are violated. In helping her be a survivor, the man should assume the role of her trusted, intimate friend. Her emotional feelings and needs should be taken seriously. When she is uncomfortable or vetoes something, even a hug, her rights and personal boundaries should be respected. You should be willing to proceed at her pace, not yours. Together, you will regain comfort and confidence with intimacy and sexuality. Healing is more likely if you utilize the services of a therapist rather than proceeding on your own.

Touch—whether affectionate, sensual, or sexual—is voluntary, mutual, pleasure-oriented. Healing from rape centers around "living well is the best revenge." The rapist no longer controls your self-esteem or sexuality. Rape is the opposite of intimacy. Regaining desire, arousal, orgasm, and satisfaction is one component of healing from a rape experience, but not the central one. The core is regaining a sense of personal integrity, trust in herself and her intimate relationship, and feeling pride in being a survivor. You play an integral role in the healing process.

CLOSING THOUGHTS

Traditionally, male sexual trauma has been ignored and minimized. This is not acceptable. Males who have been sexually abused need to confront it with support from friends, family, spouse, and community so they can be proud survivors, not silent victims.

Males with noxious paraphilias like pedophiles, who engage in incestuous behavior, or rape need to be confronted and the harmful behavior eliminated. Males deny these are destructive behaviors and minimize the damage to victims. Crisis intervention and ongoing therapy programs help victims learn to be survivors and retake control of their personal and sexual lives. However, the best treatment is prevention. It is the male's responsibility to confront and break the pattern of abusive and coercive sexual behavior. The sexually abusive male can change his destructive sexual behavior, and needs to seek competent treatment. If not, legal remedies must be enforced to stop these sexual patterns. There needs to be an individual and cultural commitment which recognizes male sexuality cannot be expressed in ways which involve force, coercion, or harm to others. Males need to be active supporters of spouses, children, and friends who have been sexually victimized. Although therapy is helpful, and usually necessary, the man cannot abdicate his responsibility to be a caring, involved spouse or parent. He is an active partner in healing.

EPILOGUE

We live in a time of rapidly changing sexual attitudes, behaviors, and norms. Ideas and values that were taken for granted as recently as ten years ago (when the first edition of this book was published) are no longer valid. Attitudes toward male sexuality are among those which have undergone the greatest change. Men used to be very certain of their place in the world. They occupied the most important positions; they were the decision makers, the leaders. In the domestic realm, the man was supreme. Patriarchy was the most common family structure.

Male dominance was particularly strong in sexual relationships. Men were considered to have a greater need for sex, a greater knowledge of sex, and to have enjoyed sex more. The woman's duty was to follow the male's lead. Even the sexual position that enjoyed (and enjoys) the greatest popularity—male on top—stressed male dominance. The theme was the man wanted and needed sex, it was the woman who said no. The sexual double standard did not end premaritally but extended through marriage and into extramarital relationships.

All this is changing. There are holdouts, of course—both men and women who cling to the double standard, who want the old male-centered domestic and sexual hierarchy to endure. These traditionalists are fighting a losing battle. Sexual equity is one of the building principles of today's world and will continue to be in the future. In business, politics, interpersonal relations, and in sex, women are demanding the equity that has for so long been denied them. The research evidence is clear—intellectually, behaviorally, emotionally, and sexually there are many more similarities than differences between men and women. Equity is the goal that couples and the culture are striving for.

As men, we ought to rejoice that this is finally happening. The double standard was never really in our interest. It emphasized what was different in the emotional and sexual responses of men and women rather than what was similar. Under the double standard, we believed the man's only goal was intercourse and orgasm. Everything else was superfluous. Women, on the other hand, were supposed to care about gentle caresses, intimacy, and integrated sexuality. It was as if men and women were two entirely different species or, as the popular, but misleading, psychology book said, "from different planets."

With the decline of the double standard and the increase in scientific research into human sexuality, it is increasingly clear that men and women have similar psychological, sexual and intimacy needs. Men find gentleness, sensual awareness, and intimacy greatly enhance their sexual and psychological well-being. Women find their potential for genital response, capacity for orgasm, and sexual desire are as great as men's. Some men find the idea of a woman who is sexually active and responsive threatening, a demand for sexual performance rather than an invitation to share sexual pleasure. A far healthier attitude is to celebrate the fact that men and women, after so many years of alienation, have an opportunity to develop a respectful, cooperative, trusting, and satisfying emotional and sexual relationship. Having discovered their intimacy and sexual needs are similar, they can now collaborate on finding the best ways of fulfilling them.

We hope this book has increased sexual awareness and understanding. A plethora of publications have been devoted to awakening women to the aspects of their sexuality that have for too long been ignored. There has been a paucity of similar works directed at men. Our aim has been to provide accurate information on male sexuality and to influence men to become sensually aware, responsible for their sexuality, able to communicate sexual feelings and preferences, conscious of the role sexuality plays throughout their lives, and integrate sexuality with their personal, emotional, and family lives. Such changes may seem like a lot to ask for, and yet, there are few areas in which there are such powerful incentives for change.

It is in a man's—any man's—best interest to make the transition from sexual performance machine to sexual person. By doing so, he can increase not only his sexual pleasure but his level of satisfaction with himself, his spouse, family, and life in general. It is time we realize what a positive element sexuality can be and how we can use it to make our relationships and lives more rewarding.

APPENDIX I
CHOOSING A THERAPIST

As stated at the beginning, this is not a do-it-yourself therapy book. Men are reluctant to consult a therapist, feeling to do so is a sign of "craziness," inadequacy, that their life is out of control, or their relationship is in dire straits. Actually, seeking professional help is a sign of psychological strength. Entering individual, sex, or marital therapy means you realize there is a problem and have made a commitment to resolving the problem.

The mental health field is confusing. Individual psychotherapy, sex therapy, and marital therapy are offered by several types of professionals, including psychologists, social workers, marriage therapists, psychiatrists, sex therapists, and pastoral counselors. The background of the practitioner is of less importance than his competence in dealing with your specific problem.

Many people have health insurance that provides coverage for mental health, and thus can afford the services of a private practitioner. Those who do not have either the financial resources or insurance could consider a city or county mental health clinic, a university or medical school mental health outpatient clinic, or a family services center. Clinics usually have a sliding-fee scale: the fee is based on your ability to pay.

In choosing a therapist, be assertive in asking about credentials and areas of expertise. Ask the clinician how long therapy can be expected to last and whether there is a focus on communication, problem solving, emotional issues, and/or sexual problems. If you are seeking marital therapy, ask how many of his couples stay together and how many divorce. A competent therapist will not object to discussing these issues. Be especially diligent in questioning credentials, such as university degrees and licenses, of people who call themselves personal counselors, marriage counselors, or sex counselors. There are poorly qualified persons—and some outright quacks—in any field.

One of the best resources for obtaining a referral is to call a local professional organization such as a psychological association, marriage and family therapy association, mental health association, or mental health clinic. You can ask for a referral from a family physician, minister, or friend. If you are experiencing a sexual problem, you can contact the American Association of Sex Educators, Counselors, and Therapists, P.O. Box 238, Mount Vernon, IA 52314, (319) 895-8407 for a list of certified sex therapists in your area.

Feel free to talk with two or three therapists before deciding on one with whom to work. Be aware of comfort with the therapist, degree of rapport, and whether the therapist's assessment of the problem and approach to treatment make sense to you. Once you begin therapy, give it a chance to be helpful. There are few miracle cures. Change requires commitment and is a gradual and often difficult process. Although some people benefit from short-term therapy (fewer than ten sessions), most people find the therapeutic process will take four months to a year. The role of the therapist is that of a consultant rather than decision maker. Therapy requires effort, both in the session and at home. Therapy focuses on changing attitudes, feelings, and behavior, which improves self-esteem and makes your sexual life and relationship more satisfying.

APPENDIX II
BOOKS FOR FURTHER READING

Bing, Elizabeth and Libby Coleman, *Making Love During Pregnancy*, New York, Bantam Books, 1983.

Butler, Robert and Myrna Lewis, *Love and Sex After Sixty*, New York, Ballantine, 1993.

Castleman, Michael, *Sexual Solutions*, New York, Simon and Schuster, 1989.

Gordon, Sol, *Why Love Is Not Enough*, Holbrook, MA, Bob Adams, 1990.

Gottman, John, *Why Marriages Succeed or Fail*, New York, Simon and Schuster, 1994.

Levinson, Daniel, *Seasons of a Man's Life*, New York, Knopf, 1978.

Maltz, Wendy, *The Sexual Healing Journey*, New York, HarperCollins, 1991.

McCarthy, Barry and Emily McCarthy, *Sexual Awareness*, New York, Carroll and Graf, 1993.

———, *Confronting The Victim Role*, New York, Carroll and Graf, 1993.

———, *Intimate Marriage*, New York, Carroll and Graf, 1992.

———, *Couple Sexual Awareness*, New York, Carroll and Graf, 1990.

———, *Female Sexual Awareness*, New York, Carroll and Graf, 1989.

Michael, Robert, John Gagnon, Edward Laumann, and Gina Kolata, *Sex in America*, Boston, Little, Brown, 1994.

Notarius, Cliff and Howard Markman, *We Can Work It Out,* New York, Putnam, 1993.

Zilbergeld, Bernie, *The New Male Sexuality,* New York, Bantam Books, 1992.

APPENDIX III
SOURCE NOTES

The field of human sexuality is based on scientific studies, but the data is not as reliable, valid, and representative as would be desired. This is due partly to the difficulty in obtaining funding for research is this value-laden, controversial area and partly due to changes in sexual attitudes, behavior, and values. The following sources provide the best estimates of peoples' sexual behavior.

1. Kinsey, A., Pomeroy, W. & Martin, C., *Sexual Behavior in the Human Male,* Philadelphia, Saunders, 1948.
2. Kinsey, A., Pomeroy, W., Martin, C. & Gebhard, P., *Sexual Behavior in the Human Female,* Philadelphia, Saunders, 1953.
3. Masters, W. & Johnson, V., *Human Sexual Response,* Boston, Little, Brown, 1966.
4. Masters, W. & Johnson, V., *Human Sexual Inadequacy,* Boston, Little, Brown, 1970.
5. Michael, R., Gagnon, J., Laumann, E. & Kolata, G., *Sex in America,* Boston, Little, Brown. 1997.
6. The Institute of Medicine, *The Hidden Epidemic: Confronting Sexually Transmitted Diseases,* Washington, D.C., National Academy Press, 1996.
7. Reinish, T., *The Kinsey Institute New Report on Sex,* New York, St. Martin's, 1990.
8. Hatcher, R., *Contraceptive Technology,* New York, Irvington, 1996.
9. Butler, K. & Lewis, M., *Love and Sex After Sixty,* New York, Ballantine, 1993.

10. Leiblum, S. & Rosen, R., *Sexual Desire Disorders,* New York, Guilford, 1988.
11. Laumann, E., Gagnon, J., Michael, R. & Michaels, S., *The Social Organization of Sexuality,* Chicago, University of Chicago, 1994.
12. Metz, M., Pryor, J., Nesvacic, L., Abuzzahab, F. & Koznar, J., "Premature Ejaculation," *Journal of Sex and Marital Therapy,* 1997, 23, 3-24.
13. Rosen, R. & Leiblum, S., *Erectile Disorders,* New York, Guildford, 1992.
14. Smith, T., *The Demography of Sexual Behavior,* Menlo Park, CA, Kaiser Family Foundation, 1994.
15. Martin, T & Bumpass, L., "Recent Trends in Marital Disruption," *Demography,* 1989, 26, 37-51.
16. Laumann, E., Gagnon, J., Michael, R. & Michaels, S., *The Socialization of Sexuality,* Chicago, University of Chicago, 1994.
17. Finkelhor, D., *Sexually Victimized Children,* New York, Free Press, 1979.